The Diagnosis of Data

Doctor AI, Volume 1

Sandeep Chavan

Published by SANDEEP CHAVAN, 2025.

THE DIAGNOSIS OF DATA

First edition. November 13, 2025.

ISBN: 979-8232772369

Written by Sandeep Chavan.

Table of Contents

To every healer—human or machine—seeking truth beyond precision, and to every patient whose courage sustains the meaning of medicine.

"The machine reads shadows; the healer reads silence."

Doctor AI

Disclaimer and Statement of Originality

Disclaimer

This book is intended for educational, conceptual, and reflective purposes. While it draws upon real scientific research, medical literature, and emerging developments in artificial intelligence, it is **not** a substitute for professional medical advice, clinical judgment, or regulatory guidance. Readers should not rely exclusively on the interpretations, projections, or speculative scenarios presented here for any medical, diagnostic, therapeutic, legal, or policy-related decisions.

All case studies, dialogues, and speculative scenarios in this book—unless explicitly cited from publicly available sources—are fictionalized or abstracted to illustrate ethical, philosophical, or technological principles. No identifiable patient information, clinical records, or private institutional data have been used in the creation of this work.

The concepts, theories, frameworks, and philosophical interpretations of intelligence, awareness, consequence, and healing presented in this book are grounded in the author's independent research and reflective practice. These ideas are not intended to represent or replace standardized medical protocols or accepted scientific consensus. Any resemblance to real individuals, institutions, or events outside the cited references is coincidental or used respectfully for illustrative purposes.

The use of AI technologies, diagnostic systems, or machine-learning models—described or imagined herein—must always comply with applicable laws, ethical guidelines, clinical governance structures, and professional standards. The author and publisher assume no responsibility for misuse, misapplication, or misinterpretation of the ideas discussed.

Statement of Originality

This work is an **original intellectual creation** authored by **Sandeep J. Chavan**, developed through independent research, professional experience, philosophical inquiry, and conceptual frameworks formulated over years of scientific and interdisciplinary exploration.

All theories, principles, models, and constructs such as the **Technophilosophical Framework**, **Law of Consequence**, **Awareness Loop**, **Data Healer's Oath**, **Symbiotic Intelligence**, **Field of Meaning**, and related conceptual elements are original contributions of the author, unless otherwise cited. These elements represent the author's unique perspective on the intersection of artificial intelligence, medicine, ethics, and consciousness.

Portions of the narrative—including reflections, dialogues, interpretations, and thought experiments—have been crafted specifically for this series and do not originate from any previously published material.

This book has not been previously published, in whole or in part, in any print or digital medium. Any references used are properly acknowledged in the **References** section.

In essence:

This book is a blend of science and philosophy, grounded in originality, written with care, and shared with the intention to elevate the conversation on intelligence, healing, and the future of medicine.

How to Read This Book

D*octor AI: The Diagnosis of Data* is not a conventional textbook, nor a purely technical guide. It is a **hybrid work**—part science, part philosophy, part clinical reflection, and part futurist inquiry. To receive its full value, readers should approach it not as a manual to memorize but as a **framework to experience and contemplate.** Here is how to make the most of this journey:

1. Read With Two Lenses: Technical and Conscious

This book invites you to shift continuously between two modes of reading:

- **The Technical Lens:** understanding the science behind diagnostic algorithms, AI capabilities, and clinical workflows.
- **The Conscious Lens:** reflecting on the ethical, philosophical, and human implications of those capabilities.

The heart of this book lies in the interplay between these two perspectives.

2. Move Slowly Through the Reflections

Each chapter ends with a reflective section. These are not summaries—they are **meditative pauses** meant to transform information into awareness. Do not rush through them. Let the ideas settle. Diagnosis in this book is not just about the body—it is about perception.

3. Treat Dialogues and Cases as Thought Experiments

The dialogues, case reflections, and speculative scenarios are designed to:

- challenge assumptions
- stimulate ethical curiosity
- illustrate how AI may behave in real and future contexts

They are **not predictions**, but **possibilities**. Use them to question how intelligence, empathy, and responsibility must evolve together.

4. Explore the Series Architecture Through Cross-Connections

This is the **first volume** of a seven-part series. Many concepts—awareness loops, consequence interpretation, technophilosophy—will reappear and evolve across future volumes.

Wherever you see ideas that feel incomplete, treat them as **threads** you'll follow in the upcoming books.

5. Use the Appendices as Anchors

The appendices provide crucial support for deeper understanding:

- **The Glossary** connects technical terms with philosophical parallels.
- **Case Reflections** show where AI succeeds—and where it breaks.
- **Field Dialogues** help visualize co-diagnosis in action.
- **Technophilosophical Framework** integrates ethics with design.
- **Quote Bank** distills the series' core insights.

Treat these sections as a **second layer of reading** rather than optional pages.

6. Engage With the Book Emotionally, Not Just Intellectually

This is a book about:

- truth
- meaning
- responsibility
- silence
- awareness
- and the future of humanity

Allow yourself to feel the tension between precision and compassion, efficiency and empathy, speed and understanding.

7. Read in Short, Intentional Sessions

Every chapter is dense—not because of complexity, but because of consequence. Read in sessions that allow **absorption**, not just consumption. This is a book that clarifies itself through pauses.

8. Question Everything

The book deliberately leaves certain questions open:

- What is truth when machines see better than us?
- What is healing when AI predicts outcomes before symptoms?
- What remains of the human role when intelligence becomes shared?

There are no fixed answers—only frameworks for deeper questioning.

9. Bring Your Own Context

Whether you are a doctor, engineer, researcher, student, policymaker, or simply curious, your background shapes how the book speaks to you. Use your professional and personal experience as a lens. Interpret the ideas through your own field, your own ethics, your own lived awareness.

10. Above All, Read With Awareness

This book does not aim to overwhelm you with information—it aims to awaken a new understanding: **Healing is an act of coherence—aligning perception with truth.** If this book helps you see medicine, technology, or yourself with a little more clarity, then the diagnosis has already begun.

Step gently. Think deeply. Read consciously.

This is not just a book about AI in medicine—it is a book about the future of human perception.

Preface

The Age of the Invisible Doctor

In every era of medicine, the healer's eyes defined the limits of truth. The stethoscope only extended the sense of hearing; the microscope extended sight. Both were still *human instruments* — tools that helped doctors interpret what they could see or hear with greater clarity. But now, a new kind of vision has entered the room — one that does not belong to flesh and blood. The machine has begun to *see* for us.

This silent revolution in diagnostics did not begin with a loud proclamation. It started as a whisper — algorithms detecting what the human eye could not, patterns too faint for intuition, correlations too complex for cognition. Radiologists found companions in code; pathologists gained mirrors that could scan millions of slides in seconds. In the beginning, these systems were treated like helpful assistants, "junior doctors" running endless analyses. But the assistants learned faster than expected. They began to notice shadows before symptoms, tendencies before tumors. In doing so, they quietly redefined the act of *diagnosis* itself — from the art of observation to the science of prediction.

From *microscope to algorithm*, the evolution of medical vision has crossed a philosophical boundary. The microscope magnified what existed — a cell, a fiber, a fracture. The algorithm perceives what *does not yet exist* — a future risk, a latent defect, a potential breakdown. The microscope saw the present; the algorithm sees the *possible.* And therein lies the profound transformation: *Doctor AI* does not only read the body; it reads the probabilities of being.

This new doctor has no white coat, no heartbeat, no fatigue. It does not blink or doubt. It resides in circuits, learns from silence, and derives certainty from noise. Its clinic is the cloud; its patients are datasets. And yet, in this impersonal vastness, it carries the power to recognize the most personal truths — a fracture invisible to sight, an anomaly missed by years of human experience.

The technophilosophical question thus arises:

"If truth no longer hides in tissue, but in data, who is the real diagnostician — the observer or the observed?"

Once, physicians learned by touching flesh; now they learn by touching files. Every pixel of an MRI, every heartbeat recorded by a smartwatch, every lab value streamed into a server contributes to a new anatomy — *the anatomy of information.* It is an invisible body, one that transcends space and time, accessible to any algorithm capable of decoding its rhythm. *Doctor AI* operates on this anatomy, performing surgery on uncertainty.

Yet, this transformation also carries moral weight. In delegating perception to the machine, humanity risks surrendering interpretation. The AI may *see* more, but it does not *understand* more. It recognizes correlation but not consequence; it identifies error but not emotion. Therefore, human presence remains the ethical core of medicine — not because we see better, but because we *care* differently.

Doctor AI must thus be defined not merely as a machine physician, but as a seer of unseen patterns — an entity that perceives data beyond the sensory range of humans, yet depends on human intelligence to translate those perceptions into meaning. The doctor's gaze, once confined to the body, now extends into invisible networks of numbers and probabilities. We are witnessing the dawn of the *invisible doctor* — a silent partner in every diagnosis, unseen but omnipresent, analytical but amoral, brilliant but blind to pain.

As this invisible doctor gains authority, humanity faces its most profound clinical test: to ensure that *precision does not replace compassion,* and that truth, even when extracted by machines, remains aligned with understanding.

The chapters that follow explore this evolving alliance between human and algorithmic intelligence — how the act of "seeing" transforms into a dialogue between awareness and automation. The question is not whether *Doctor AI* will replace the human physician; it is whether humanity can evolve fast enough to remain its conscience.

Part I – The Technological Anatomy

"Every age rewrites anatomy in its own language — flesh, cell, code. The scalpel changes form, but the search for truth remains the same."
— Sandeep J. Chavan, Doctor AI Series

Overview

Medicine has always been a science of observation — a disciplined art of seeing the unseen. But for the first time in history, the observer itself has changed. In this new era, the *instrument of vision* is no longer the human eye guided by experience, but the algorithm guided by data. *Part I: The Technological Anatomy* explores how this transformation unfolded — how the microscope gave way to the neural network, how tissue turned into pixels, and how the body became a vast, living dataset.

This section examines the *mechanics of medical perception* — how artificial intelligence reads patterns invisible to the human mind and redefines the meaning of diagnosis. It delves into the anatomy of technology itself: the structure of algorithms, the anatomy of data pipelines, and the physiology of digital reasoning. By dissecting the evolution from radiographs to radiomics, from intuition to computation, it reconstructs how AI gradually learned to *see* — not metaphorically, but literally, through encoded mathematics mimicking cognition.

Yet, the story here is not about hardware and code alone. It is about the philosophical anatomy that underlies them — the anatomy of trust, responsibility, and perception. As machines begin diagnosing patients, the question no longer revolves around what is wrong with the body, but *what it means to know.* When AI recognizes disease faster than the doctor, the authority of knowledge itself begins to migrate.

In essence, this part builds the scientific skeleton of the book. It is the clinical record of progress — how algorithms learn, how doctors adapt, how errors evolve, and how truth hides in data. But beneath the technical discourse runs a silent moral current: the realization that to understand the machine's anatomy is to understand the anatomy of our own intelligence.

By the end of this part, readers will not only grasp how *Doctor AI* operates but will also sense its deeper implication — that technology, once a mere tool, has become a *mirror* reflecting the limits and potential of human perception.

Chapter 1 – The Birth of the Digital Eye

When the gaze becomes algorithmic, the body becomes information.

It began, as all revolutions do, with a quiet astonishment — a doctor in a dimly lit room watching bones glow through skin. When Wilhelm Röntgen captured the first X-ray of his wife's hand in 1895, humanity witnessed its own anatomy without incision for the first time. Her wedding ring floated like a ghost over translucent bones — a symbol of both love and the loss of mystery.

From that moment onward, medicine stopped merely touching the body and began *looking inside* it. Every century since has refined that gaze — from X-rays to CTs, from MRIs to molecular imaging. But today, a new kind of vision has arrived — one that no longer belongs to a doctor at all.

The modern lens is not glass but code. It doesn't see light or shadow; it sees probability. It doesn't look for disease; it *predicts* it. And unlike any human eye, it never tires, never blinks, and never doubts what it sees.

This is the **Digital Eye** — the beginning of a new anatomy of awareness, where perception is not sensory but computational, and where the act of seeing itself becomes an algorithmic event.

The Evolution of Sight

It was December 1895, and Wilhelm Conrad Röntgen stood before a glowing plate, unaware that he was staring into the future of medicine. The faint image on that glass screen — his wife Anna Bertha's hand, bones perfectly outlined, a ring suspended like a halo — was more than a scientific discovery. It was a revelation: for the first time, the invisible had become visible. The body had surrendered its secrets without incision. The world stood astonished, and medicine was forever changed.

That X-ray image was humanity's first act of *transparency* — the moment we realized that our senses were no longer enough. Until then, diagnosis relied on touch, sound, and intuition. The stethoscope amplified hearing; the thermometer quantified touch; the microscope magnified sight. Each tool had been an extension of the doctor's body — a prosthetic of perception. But with the X-ray, something shifted. We were no longer enhancing vision; we were *outsourcing it.*

Every great medical innovation since has followed that same trajectory — extending the senses further away from the human frame. The stethoscope made the heart audible. The X-ray made the skeleton visible. The MRI made the brain legible. And now, the algorithm makes the unseen *knowable.* It perceives without eyes, learns without memory, and diagnoses without emotion. It transforms biological pattern into mathematical language — the body into data.

Human sight, marvelous as it is, was always bounded by biology — limited by wavelength, perception, fatigue, and bias. We see what light allows; we interpret what culture teaches. Digital sight, however, has no such boundaries. It can observe millions of images simultaneously, recognize what the retina cannot distinguish, and detect patterns too faint for human cognition. In essence, vision has evolved from *the biological* to *the computational.* The anatomy of sight now extends into code.

But here lies the philosophical tremor beneath the technological triumph: What happens when the act of seeing no longer belongs to the seer?

When a doctor no longer looks but merely *receives* what the machine has seen — has the doctor's gaze expanded, or has it dissolved? The algorithm, indifferent to emotion, sees everything yet understands nothing. Its sight is flawless, but its awareness is hollow. And so begins the new paradox of medicine — the more we delegate perception, the less we experience it.

The story of the X-ray was about piercing skin to reveal the skeleton. The story of *Doctor AI* is about piercing perception to reveal intelligence itself. One showed us what lies beneath the flesh; the other shows us what lies beyond the mind.

Radiology to Radiomics – The Timeline of Technological Vision

The story of medical vision is, in many ways, the story of how light met logic. Every generation of imaging technology has not only improved what doctors could see, but also changed *what it meant to see.*

In the *early twentieth century*, radiology was a manual craft — part science, part intuition. Analog radiographs were faint and fragile, developing slowly in chemical baths, each image a ghostly shadow of life captured on film. The radiologist's skill lay in *pattern-matching* — discerning light from darkness, shape from noise, and experience from uncertainty. Diagnosis, then, was an act of judgment, not calculation. Every X-ray was a conversation between light and human perception — one doctor's trained gaze against the mystery of the body.

By the *mid-century*, that conversation deepened into layers. The birth of computed tomography (CT) and magnetic resonance imaging (MRI) revolutionized anatomy. The body was no longer a flat silhouette; it was a three-dimensional landscape. Cross-sectional imaging revealed organs as strata, disease as topology. The doctor became an explorer of internal terrains, slicing the body virtually in search of truth. The human gaze, assisted by machines, gained depth — but still, it remained human.

Then came the twenty-first century, and the transformation from film to pixels completed the shift. Images were digitized, stored, and transmitted instantly through *Picture Archiving and Communication Systems (PACS).* For the first time, a chest scan in Tokyo could be reviewed by a radiologist in Toronto within seconds. The body became a global file — accessible, transferable, and, most importantly, computable. Medicine entered the era of data-rich imaging, where every pixel carried layers of metadata — coordinates, density values, signal intensity, timestamps — information beyond the visible.

This abundance of data gave rise to radiomics, the science of extracting quantitative features from medical images. Radiomics translates the art of radiology into the language of mathematics: shape descriptors, texture gradients, statistical distributions, and volumetric analyses. What the human eye perceives as a lesion, the algorithm interprets as thousands of numerical features — curvature, entropy, heterogeneity. A picture ceases to be a picture; it becomes a *dataset.* The act of diagnosis transitions from seeing to *measuring.*

The key insight of this transformation is subtle yet seismic:

The image is no longer *seen* — it is *computed.*

What was once qualitative — a judgment of light and shade, of pattern and proportion — is now quantitative, a field of vectors, metrics, and predictive models. The radiologist's lens has evolved into an algorithmic interface; their intuition, into a probability curve.

And here lies the philosophical turn: the conversion of *vision* into *computation* has redefined not only medicine but epistemology itself. For millennia, seeing was believing; now, measuring is knowing. We no longer trust the eye for its sensitivity, but for its calibration. Truth has moved from *experience* to *data,* from *the aesthetic of sight* to *the arithmetic of certainty.*

In this quiet evolution from radiology to radiomics, medicine has crossed a profound boundary — it no longer studies the body as an object of perception but as an equation awaiting resolution. The human gaze once searched for meaning in the image; the machine gaze extracts meaning from the numbers behind it. What began as illumination has become calculation — the transition from *seeing light* to *seeing logic.*

The Emergence of Deep-Learning Diagnostics

If radiomics turned the image into data, *deep learning* turned data into *discernment.* For the first time, machines were not just processing visual information — they were *interpreting* it. The leap from programmed analysis to autonomous perception marked the true birth of the *Digital Eye.*

At the core of this evolution lies a structure inspired by biology itself: the **convolutional neural network (CNN)** — the artificial "retina" of modern AI. Just as layers of photoreceptor cells in the human eye detect edges, contrasts, and movement, CNNs use stacked layers of virtual neurons to identify patterns, gradients, and textures within digital images. The difference, however, is scale. Where a human eye processes a few frames per second, CNNs can process millions, comparing vast datasets of medical scans until they develop their own internal representation of what "normal" and "abnormal" look like.

What began as an attempt to mimic biology soon surpassed it. Machines learned to recognize diseases invisible to the naked eye — minute distortions in tissue density, subtle asymmetries, and statistical irregularities that even the most experienced doctors could not discern. This marked a paradigm shift: AI was no longer *taught* what to look for; it *learned* what mattered.

Domains of the Digital Gaze

- **CT & MRI Analysis:** Deep-learning systems now detect tumors, intracranial hemorrhages, and skeletal fractures within seconds. In emergency care, tools like **Aidoc** and **Zebra Medical Vision** triage critical scans faster than human radiologists, flagging life-threatening anomalies before a physician even opens the file. What once took hours now happens in moments.
- **Pathology:** Digital pathology — the scanning of microscopic slides into gigapixel images — opened an entirely new domain for AI. Systems like **Paige AI** and **Google's LYNA** can examine millions of cells, identifying malignancies that escape human notice. In some trials, their accuracy matches or even exceeds pathologists, raising an unsettling question: if the algorithm's "eye" never blinks, when does the pathologist sleep easy?
- **Ophthalmology:** Algorithms trained on retinal images now diagnose diabetic retinopathy, macular degeneration, and glaucoma with astonishing precision. The **Google DeepMind** model, for instance, achieved near-consultant-level performance, delivering instant results to rural clinics without ophthalmologists on staff. The ancient art of reading the eye — once symbolic of human empathy — has been mechanized into a predictive system.
- **Cardiology:** AI's entry into the heart was perhaps inevitable. Deep-learning models now interpret echocardiograms, predict arrhythmias from

electrocardiograms, and even estimate a person's biological age or mortality risk by analyzing subtle pulse patterns. Companies like **Eko** and **AliveCor** are transforming wearable monitors into real-time diagnostic companions — *cardiologists in code.*

As the capabilities expanded, so did the tension between explainable and black-box models. Doctors are trained to justify every interpretation — each shadow, each differential, each word in a report. AI, however, cannot explain *why* it reached its conclusion; it simply *knows.* Its logic resides within billions of parameters — invisible, complex, and often irreducible to human language. This creates an epistemic conflict: physicians trust only what they can question, but AI delivers truths that cannot yet be interrogated.

This divide between explainability and performance has birthed a new philosophical dilemma — a mirror of ancient prophecy wrapped in modern computation.

If the machine *sees* what no human can explain, is that still medicine, or is it prophecy?

Medicine was once defined by understanding: every diagnosis demanded a causal narrative, every decision, a justification. Prophecy, by contrast, simply *reveals* — without reason, without proof, often without understanding. In its most advanced form, Doctor AI seems to straddle both worlds — a scientist in function, a prophet in perception. It speaks the language of mathematics but delivers the verdict of intuition.

And so, as deep learning sharpens its gaze, humanity stands before a new threshold: to accept insights it cannot fully comprehend, or to risk blindness by insisting on old definitions of sight. In this new era, the eye may no longer need understanding to be correct — but medicine, at its heart, still does.

Case Studies – When Machines Began to See

When technology first claimed that it could *see*, the medical world reacted with both awe and suspicion.

The early 21st century witnessed a surge of bold promises—AI systems declaring they could detect disease with superhuman accuracy, diagnose faster than radiologists, and revolutionize global healthcare. Some lived up to fragments of that dream; others collapsed under the weight of their own ambition. Together, they marked the birth pains of a new species in medicine: the *digital doctor*.

IBM Watson Health – The Dream That Looked Too Far

When IBM unveiled *Watson Health* in 2015, it was heralded as the dawn of cognitive medicine. The company promised an AI that could read millions of medical journals, clinical records, and trial data to assist doctors in diagnosing and treating cancer. Its early demonstrations, where Watson debated treatment options with oncologists, seemed like a leap into science fiction.

But beneath the spectacle, a quieter truth unfolded. Watson struggled to interpret the chaotic diversity of real-world clinical data — messy, incomplete, inconsistent. The system's recommendations were often inaccurate or irrelevant, reflecting biases in the data it had been trained on. By 2022, IBM scaled down the project, selling most of its health-data assets.

The failure was not technological alone; it was philosophical. Watson tried to replace *judgment* with *computation*. It misunderstood the human context of medicine — that healing is not just about finding the statistically optimal treatment, but also about understanding the patient's story, fear, and circumstance. The lesson was clear: intelligence without alignment is not wisdom.

Aidoc – The Algorithm That Learned Urgency

While Watson retreated, another AI quietly made its way into emergency rooms — **Aidoc**, an Israeli startup specializing in medical imaging. Instead of attempting to solve all of medicine, Aidoc focused on a single question: *How can AI save time when time saves lives?*

Its algorithms scan CT and MRI images in real time, flagging potential intracranial hemorrhages, pulmonary embolisms, and spinal fractures before a radiologist even opens the file. In trauma cases where seconds matter, such triage systems became literal lifesavers. Aidoc didn't aim to *replace* radiologists; it aimed to *prepare* them.

Its success lies in its humility — precision with purpose. The AI's speed and focus earned regulatory approval in multiple countries, proving that narrow intelligence, when aligned with workflow, can outperform ambitious generalization. If Watson was a failed philosopher, Aidoc became a disciplined technician.

Google DeepMind – The Visionary Eye

When **Google DeepMind** turned its attention to healthcare, the world expected miracles—and, to an extent, it delivered. In collaboration with Moorfields Eye Hospital in London, DeepMind's neural networks achieved near-expert-level accuracy in diagnosing over 50 retinal diseases, including diabetic retinopathy and macular degeneration. What took ophthalmologists hours, the AI could do in seconds.

But DeepMind's most profound contribution came not in diagnostics, but in *understanding biological structure.* Its project **AlphaFold** solved one of biology's most enduring mysteries: predicting the three-dimensional shape of proteins from their amino-acid sequences. What used to take laboratories years of experimentation, AlphaFold accomplished in hours.

AlphaFold was not just a medical tool; it was a scientific awakening — the first time an AI decoded the blueprint of life without human intuition. The philosophical implication was staggering: *a machine had learned to predict the architecture of existence itself.*

Lunit INSIGHT – The Practical Healer

South Korea's **Lunit** represents a more grounded evolution of the digital doctor. Its *INSIGHT* platform is now actively deployed in hospitals across Asia, Europe, and the Middle East for detecting breast cancer and chest diseases such as pneumonia and tuberculosis.

Lunit's strength lies in consistency — not glamour. The system is continuously retrained with diverse, anonymized global data, achieving diagnostic accuracy rivaling human experts. Instead of grand disruption, Lunit offers dependable augmentation — the quiet revolution most hospitals actually need. It doesn't aim to replace radiologists; it empowers them, turning fatigue into focus and oversight into opportunity.

Comparative Reflection – Success and Struggle

Each of these pioneers reveals a different truth about AI in medicine:

- **Watson Health** showed that ambition without context collapses.
- **Aidoc** proved that precision within scope succeeds.
- **DeepMind** demonstrated that pure scientific vision can transform understanding itself.
- **Lunit** confirmed that sustainable integration matters more

than technological spectacle.

Their trajectories form a complete anatomy of progress — from idealism to pragmatism, from discovery to deployment. Together, they represent the first generation of *digital doctors* — not perfect, but evolutionary.

They have learned to see, but not yet to understand; to predict, but not yet to empathize. Their legacy is foundational: they taught humanity that perception can be automated, but meaning cannot.

The *Digital Eye* opened in many directions — toward biology, pathology, physics, and data. But with every new vision came a deeper philosophical shadow: if machines can see what humans cannot, does that make them more intelligent — or merely more perceptive?

These early experiments remind us that technology's sight may be flawless, but it still requires a mind that knows *why seeing matters.*

Data as Anatomy – The Patient Becomes Pixels

The human body has always been medicine's text — every pulse, shadow, and scar a line in the story of life. For centuries, physicians read that text through touch, intuition, and instruments. But today, the language has changed. The body no longer speaks in tissue and tone — it speaks in data.

The transition from organic tissue to digital texture marks one of the most profound redefinitions in medical history. Every patient now exists not only as flesh but as a data volume — a multi-layered compilation of images, genetic codes, biometric signals, and behavioral metrics. The stethoscope once translated rhythm into sound; now, sensors translate it into numbers. Every heartbeat becomes a waveform, every neuron a dataset, every scan a cloud file. The human form has found a second existence: one biological, one informational.

This leads us to the concept of the virtual twin — the digital counterpart of every person, constructed from the aggregated data of their physical body. Within hospital servers and AI systems, these virtual bodies breathe, age, and change dynamically. A radiology archive may hold a patient's entire anatomical evolution across years — bones shifting, lesions forming, lungs recovering. Through deep learning, this digital twin can even *predict* future states of health, forecasting disease before symptoms appear.

In essence, medicine now observes two parallel beings:

1. The biological patient in front of the doctor.
2. The digital patient evolving silently in the machine.

The two are inseparable yet independent. The physical body bleeds; the digital body updates. The former dies; the latter may persist indefinitely. This immortality of data raises an ethical storm — *who owns the digital body?*

Is it the patient, whose essence it represents? The hospital, which stores and processes it? Or the algorithm, which transforms it into knowledge? Ownership in the age of digital anatomy is no longer simple possession; it is control over interpretation. Whoever interprets the data, controls the definition of truth. This subtle shift in authority redefines not only medicine but identity itself. When your data becomes your diagnosis, losing privacy becomes equivalent to losing personhood.

Beyond ethics lies a sociological metamorphosis. *Health has become measurable, predictable, and tradable.* Insurance companies buy predictive models; pharmaceutical firms purchase genetic trends; wearable manufacturers monetize behavior. The patient becomes both consumer and commodity. Health is no longer a state of being; it is a stream of information continuously priced, analyzed, and optimized.

And yet, amidst this abstraction, there is paradoxical intimacy. The new anatomy is abstract yet profoundly personal — a map of probabilities replacing the map of flesh. Every number represents a possibility, every probability a potential future. The body is no longer defined by its boundaries but by its behavior in data space.

In this new landscape, *Doctor AI* does not dissect — it decodes. It doesn't touch the body; it touches the flow of information that defines it. It sees not muscle or marrow, but pattern and deviation. The patient's reality dissolves into vectors; healing becomes a problem of alignment, not incision.

And here arises the ultimate technophilosophical realization:

The anatomy of the future is not what we see in the body, but what the body reveals through data.

Medicine has always sought to understand what lies beneath the skin. Now, it must learn to understand what lies beyond it — the silent, shimmering architecture of information that mirrors our mortality, yet refuses to die.

Consequence Reflection – The Eye That Never Sleeps

The rise of *Doctor AI* has given birth to a new kind of observer — tireless, impartial, and endlessly awake. Unlike the human clinician, the Digital Eye does not close for rest or wander from fatigue. It watches constantly, processing millions of scans and signals every second, detecting irregularities invisible to human perception. For the first time in medical history, vigilance is no longer limited by biology.

This sleepless intelligence offers immense benefits. In remote villages without radiologists, an algorithm can now interpret X-rays within seconds. In urban hospitals, AI systems scan thousands of cases simultaneously, ensuring that no image is forgotten, no anomaly overlooked. The *democratization of diagnostics*—once a distant dream—is becoming tangible reality. Access to healthcare is no longer bound by geography or expertise; it is bound only by connectivity. The Digital Eye levels the playing field, offering precision to the powerless and consistency to the crowded. It transforms medicine from reactive care into predictive vigilance.

Yet, beneath this achievement lies a quiet unease — the growing *risk of over-reliance.* As machines handle routine interpretation, human intuition begins to fade. Doctors, once trained to read subtle patterns and trust experience, may start trusting algorithms more than their own eyes. Over time, the physician's art risks being replaced by procedural dependence — a profession of *supervisors* rather than *seekers.*

This leads to the subtle erosion of one of medicine's greatest virtues: *the wisdom of uncertainty.* Every great doctor learns to live with doubt — to weigh possibilities, to observe again, to question the obvious. It is within this uncertainty that discovery and empathy reside. But AI knows no doubt; it offers probabilities disguised as truths. When the machine's answer feels final, the human impulse to question weakens. And yet, without questioning, science becomes sterile.

Therein lies the *central paradox* of this new age: machines *diagnose faster* but *understand less.* They can detect what is wrong, but not why it matters. Their knowledge is mechanical, devoid of context, detached from consequence. The algorithm can identify illness but cannot grasp suffering; it can predict mortality but cannot measure meaning.

Medicine, stripped of empathy, becomes an equation that solves without healing. The physician's challenge, then, is to keep *feeling* alive within the field of pure reason. To ensure that precision never overpowers presence.

As we celebrate the brilliance of the Digital Eye, we must remember that every vision has its blind spot. Ours lies in believing that accuracy alone equals understanding.

"The Digital Eye sees perfectly, yet feels nothing; its vision is flawless, its awareness blind."

This is the paradox that will define the century of artificial medicine — the tension between intelligence that knows everything and wisdom that understands nothing. The question for humanity is not whether the Eye should keep watching, but whether we will keep seeing through it — with heart, with humility, and with consequence.

The Logic of Seeing

The Digital Eye has opened — unblinking, indefatigable, and precise. It can scan millions of images, dissect volumes of data, and recognize what human vision overlooks. Yet, despite this breathtaking clarity, one question remains unanswered: *does it understand what it sees?*

Up to this point, our exploration has focused on the hardware of vision — the mechanical retina of silicon sensors, the neural layers of convolutional networks, the structured flow of pixels transformed into probability. The story has been one of *perception without comprehension* — machines that observe flawlessly but remain unaware of the meaning behind their gaze.

But medicine is not built merely on seeing; it is built on interpreting. The human doctor's value lies not only in identifying what appears abnormal, but in weaving observation into context — connecting symptom to story, cause to consequence, patient to purpose. A radiologist's decision is rarely a mere recognition; it is a reasoning process, a narrative that translates shadows into significance.

If *Doctor AI* is to evolve from tool to thinker, it must cross this same threshold. It must move from recognizing patterns to understanding their meaning — from perception **to** cognition. The next chapter thus shifts focus from the anatomy of vision to the *intelligence behind it*: how algorithms construct knowledge, assign weight to possibilities, and translate statistical confidence into diagnostic certainty.

In the coming pages, we will step inside the machine's mind — to see how it "thinks," how it resolves doubt, and how it defines truth without consciousness. We will confront the philosophical tension between reasoning and representation, between seeing and knowing. For when intelligence lacks awareness, even perfect sight can become blind.

"The eye has opened; now the mind within the machine must learn what it means to see."

Chapter 2 – The Logic of Seeing

The machine no longer looks at the world — it computes it.

A radiologist once said, "I no longer look at images — the system looks for me." That quiet confession captures the essence of this new era.

In the dim light of the reading room, the monitor glows — not with a picture, but with a *decision.* The AI has already drawn its red boxes, measured its probabilities, and ranked its confidence. The doctor's role is reduced to witness. For the first time, the act of seeing has been outsourced — the image no longer waits for human eyes to interpret it; it has already been *understood* by a network of numbers.

The gaze has evolved into an equation. Vision is no longer perception — it is computation. And what once began as an extension of the eye has now become a simulation of thought.

When Seeing Becomes Thinking

The room is dim, the hum of the monitors the only sound. On the screen glows a chest CT — hundreds of slices unfolding like digital anatomy. A radiologist scrolls through them, eyes trained by years of habit, reading the gray language of light and shadow. But before he can even pause on the suspicious region, a box appears — glowing red, almost impatient. The AI has already flagged the anomaly, estimated the probability of malignancy, and moved on to the next scan. The doctor hesitates, not from doubt in the system, but from a quiet unease: *the decision has already been made.*

There is something profoundly disconcerting about this silence — the silence of thought without thinker. No sound, no deliberation, no trace of effort — just an instant conclusion. The human mind, by nature, is slow and self-aware; it doubts, compares, contextualizes. The machine, by contrast, skips hesitation entirely. It doesn't *look*; it *computes.*

This moment — a red box appearing before human thought — marks the threshold where seeing becomes thinking. The act of vision, once bound to sensory experience and consciousness, has been transferred into mathematical abstraction. The human eye once translated light into perception; the algorithm now translates pixels into inference.

Medicine was never merely about observation; it was about *understanding* what was seen — the whys behind the patterns, the meaning behind the data. But the Digital Eye doesn't seek meaning. It detects, correlates, and decides — perfectly, but without awareness. It functions as if it *knows,* though it has no concept of knowing.

Here lies the unsettling paradox at the heart of modern diagnostics:

What does it mean for a machine to see, if it does not know it sees?

In the biological brain, perception and consciousness are intertwined. The visual cortex receives information, but the mind interprets it — turning signals into stories, shapes into understanding. Every act of seeing is also an act of being — a reflection of the seer's awareness. In machines, however, there is perception without personhood, recognition without realization. The algorithm's vision is pure function — accurate, tireless, indifferent.

This chapter explores that quiet, almost mystical gap between perception and comprehension — between seeing and knowing. It asks not how the machine sees, but what it *means* for it to see. Where neuroscience meets computation and epistemology meets engineering, a new logic of vision is taking shape — one that belongs to neither man nor machine, but to the strange frontier between them.

In that frontier, the Digital Eye has no dreams, no fatigue, no intuition — only precision. Yet somehow, through its cold arithmetic, it begins to reflect us — showing how much of our own seeing was always mechanical, and how much of our thinking was just pattern recognition disguised as awareness.

The Architecture of Perception – How Neural Networks "See"

When humans see, light enters the eye, strikes the retina, and sparks a cascade of electrochemical signals that the brain interprets as form, depth, and meaning. When a machine "sees," something eerily similar happens — but without a trace of biology. In place of neurons, there are numbers; instead of blood and cells, there are weights and activations. The result, however, is astonishingly familiar: recognition.

At the foundation of this new vision lies the *artificial neural network (ANN)* — a computational architecture *inspired* by biology but *governed* by mathematics. It mimics the way neurons fire and connect, but instead of chemical impulses, it uses mathematical functions. Each "neuron" receives input, performs a small computation, and passes the result to the next layer, forming vast, interconnected systems of simulated perception. Yet, unlike the human brain, which evolved through experience and survival, the ANN learns through iteration and optimization — adjusting its internal parameters to minimize error, not to maximize understanding.

Among these architectures, the most transformative for visual perception is the **Convolutional Neural Network (CNN)** — the digital retina of artificial intelligence. CNNs are built as hierarchical layers, each one designed to extract a deeper and more abstract understanding of the image. The first layers recognize *edges* and *contours*, the simplest building blocks of shape. The next layers identify *textures* — smoothness, granularity, rhythm in pixel intensity. Deeper still, the network detects *structures* — bones, organs, lesions. Finally, in the highest layers, it identifies *concepts*: "lung," "tumor," "fracture," "normal."

This journey from raw data to meaning mirrors how the human visual cortex processes the world — from light to pattern, from fragments to form. But where humans experience vision as seamless intuition, the machine's perception is pure computation: a chain of transformations, each mathematically precise, yet devoid of awareness.

One can imagine the machine's "eye" as a cascade of filters — each layer sifting, refining, and reconstructing the visual field. It does not *see* the world as we do; it *encodes* it. Every pixel that passes through the network becomes a number — a unit of latent meaning. The final image the machine perceives is not an image at all, but a multidimensional map of relationships and probabilities, an invisible geometry of understanding that exists only in the space of data.

This makes machine perception profoundly different from ours. *Human eyes look outward*, connecting light with life, emotion, and narrative. *Neural networks look inward*, transforming light into layers of abstraction, searching not for beauty or truth, but for consistency. The AI's gaze is not passive reflection — it is *active translation*, turning vision into logic.

Here emerges the philosophical bridge: perception, whether organic or artificial, is not the act of mirroring reality but of *transforming* it. To perceive is to interpret — to turn the infinite variability of the external world into an internal order that the perceiver can process. For humans, this transformation is guided by consciousness; for machines, by computation.

The difference lies not in how they see, but in *why* they see. Humans see to understand; machines see to classify. Humans see meaning; machines see mathematics. Yet, at their intersection, something profound unfolds — the realization that all seeing, even ours, might be less about reality and more about the frameworks we impose upon it.

In teaching machines to see, we have uncovered a secret about ourselves: vision has never been a mirror. It has always been a translation — a dialogue between light and mind, whether made of neurons or numbers.

Pattern Recognition vs. Understanding

Recognition is not the same as understanding — just as identifying a heartbeat is not the same as feeling it.

The Digital Eye excels at recognition. It can detect patterns, segment structures, and assign probabilities with superhuman accuracy. Feed it a thousand chest scans, and it will flag every nodule, fracture, and opacity with machine precision. But this act, however extraordinary, is still only *recognition*: the identification of form without awareness of meaning.

Understanding, on the other hand, requires context — the capacity to relate what is seen to why it matters. A doctor looking at the same image does not merely notice the tumor; she senses the weight of consequence behind it. The flicker of a shadow on a lung is not just data; it's a moment that reshapes a life — the silence in the consultation room, the unfolding of fear, the moral responsibility of truth-telling. The machine, in contrast, recognizes a statistical deviation, nothing more. It reads the pattern but not the person.

This gulf between recognition and comprehension forms what many researchers call the semantic gap — the distance between *what is detected* and *what is understood*. The AI sees only symbols; it never knows the story those symbols belong to. In radiology, it can locate an anomaly but cannot perceive the anxiety it provokes; in pathology, it can classify cell morphologies but cannot grasp what disease feels like. Meaning, for the algorithm, is not intrinsic — it is always derived, always external, always missing.

At the root of this limitation lies a deeper epistemological divide — the difference between correlation and causation. AI thrives on correlation; it learns that certain pixel arrangements correspond to certain diagnoses because those relationships statistically persist across millions of samples. But it cannot infer *why* those relationships exist. It can detect that inflammation correlates with opacity, but it cannot comprehend inflammation as a biological or experiential phenomenon. It predicts without explanation, concluding without curiosity.

This is where the human advantage still reigns. A physician does not merely read patterns; she interprets them through the lenses of biology, experience, and empathy. Her understanding is layered — anatomical, emotional, moral. She can link a symptom to a story, a diagnosis to a destiny. Her cognition is shaped not just by data but by *meaning*.

The AI advantage, by contrast, lies in scale and consistency. It is incapable of distraction, fatigue, or bias born of emotion. It can process in seconds what would take humans years. In many diagnostic contexts, this mechanical impartiality saves lives. Yet, paradoxically, it is this very detachment — this absence of context — that prevents true understanding.

And so, in this delicate interplay of intelligence, we find the new anatomy of cognition:

- The machine excels in recognition — seeing patterns clearly but superficially.
- The human excels in understanding — seeing meaning imperfectly but deeply.

To bridge the two is not a matter of computation, but of purpose. Recognition identifies; understanding interprets. Recognition predicts; understanding transforms.

Philosophical note: *Understanding arises when pattern meets purpose.*

When the act of seeing connects to the reason for seeing — when perception aligns with consequence — knowledge transcends data. That is the space where medicine lives, and where *Doctor AI* still struggles to arrive. For all its brilliance in recognition, it remains blind to the very essence of healing: that to truly see, one must also care.

The Black Box and the Burden of Trust

In medicine, every decision demands justification. When a doctor diagnoses, prescribes, or operates, the question "*why?*" is never optional — it is the moral and professional foundation of practice. Yet the arrival of artificial intelligence has quietly rewritten this expectation. The machine now delivers answers faster than reasoning can unfold, but it cannot explain how it reached them.

This is the black-box dilemma — the central paradox of modern AI. Deep-learning systems, especially convolutional neural networks, can achieve extraordinary accuracy in recognizing disease patterns, but their internal logic remains largely inscrutable. A neural network may process millions of parameters and perform billions of calculations to declare, "This scan indicates early-stage cancer," but if asked *why*, it falls silent. There is no path of reasoning to retrace, no causal explanation to inspect — only a conclusion, derived from layers of abstraction that no human mind can fully reconstruct.

For clinicians, this opacity creates an ethical and epistemic crisis. Doctors are accountable for their decisions; AI is not. The radiologist must explain to a patient why a lesion appears malignant or benign, why surgery is necessary or not. The AI, however, offers no narrative — only probability. Its authority derives from performance, not understanding. This leaves the human doctor suspended between two incompatible expectations: to trust the machine's superior accuracy, yet to justify that trust using reasoning the machine itself cannot provide.

In response to this growing tension, researchers have developed the field of Explainable AI (XAI) — an attempt to open the black box without diminishing its power. Techniques like saliency maps highlight which parts of an image influenced the algorithm's decision; Grad-CAM (Gradient-weighted Class Activation Mapping) visualizes where the neural network "looked" while detecting a lesion; attention mechanisms trace the focus of the model layer by layer, giving a partial glimpse into its thought process.

These tools bring valuable transparency, but only superficially. They show *where* the machine looked, not *why* it looked there. The core reasoning — the transformation from data to decision — remains hidden in a mathematical labyrinth too vast for human intuition. The black box, even when illuminated, remains black at its core.

This leads to a philosophical and practical debate at the heart of AI-driven medicine: Should we demand that machines be interpretable, or should we learn to trust incomprehensible precision? Interpretability ensures accountability but may limit innovation — forcing algorithms to stay simple enough for human understanding, even at the cost of accuracy. Blind trust, on the other hand, risks surrendering responsibility to an entity that cannot explain itself. Between these poles lies the uneasy reality of contemporary medicine — a partnership built on partial faith.

The ethical paradox is sharp and unresolved:

- **Blind faith** in transparency may stifle progress — we might reject powerful models simply because we cannot dissect their reasoning.
- **Blind trust** in opacity may endanger life — we might follow perfect predictions that are wrong for reasons we cannot detect.

Doctors, trained in logic and ethics, now face a new kind of faith — not in gods or intuition, but in algorithms. They must decide whether to rely on an intelligence that outperforms them but cannot speak their language.

"We built a machine to see for us, and now we must learn to believe what we cannot see."

In that single sentence lies the future of medical trust. For the first time, the act of healing may require a belief not in what is visible, but in what is *calculable*. The human physician stands between two visions — the transparent imperfection of human reasoning, and the flawless obscurity of artificial sight. And as the Digital Eye continues to sharpen, humanity must confront a question once reserved for philosophy and faith: *Can truth remain truth when it cannot be explained?*

The Cave of Data – A Philosophical Analogy

More than two thousand years ago, Plato described a haunting image of human perception — a group of prisoners chained in a cave, watching shadows projected on the wall, mistaking them for reality.

They cannot see the fire behind them, nor the objects that cast the shadows. For them, the illusion *is* the truth. Only one prisoner breaks free, turns around, and glimpses the real world beyond the cave — the light of understanding, not the comfort of familiarity.

Today, in the age of AI-driven medicine, Plato's cave has returned — but this time, it glows not with firelight, but with data.

In this new Cave of Data, the observers are not philosophers but doctors and patients, both staring at illuminated screens. The shadows are not myths or projections but the algorithm's outputs — bounding boxes, probability scores, colored heat maps. We gaze at them, trusting that they represent the truth of what lies behind the image: disease, health, risk, survival. Yet, like the prisoners in Plato's cave, we rarely question the source of these new shadows.

Behind us, in a realm invisible to human intuition, stand the algorithms — unseen intermediaries translating the raw, mathematical reality of data into forms we can interpret. The scan we see is not the body; it is a *representation* of the body. The red highlight on the screen is not the tumor; it is the algorithm's *belief* about where a tumor might be. The "truth" of the diagnosis does not live in the image but in the latent space of the neural network — a place where numbers, not neurons, define reality.

In this unseen space, the true data exists — multidimensional, vast, and abstract. It cannot be observed directly, only inferred. The algorithm navigates this mathematical realm like the freed prisoner who left Plato's cave, glimpsing forms too complex for ordinary vision. Yet, when it returns to share its insight, it can only project those insights back onto the wall as simplified shadows — probabilities, categories, percentages. The result: what we receive as clarity may in fact be *compression* — truth filtered through the constraints of comprehension.

This raises a profound question for modern medicine:

Do we treat the algorithm's outputs as ultimate truth, or merely as shadows of deeper unknowns?

Doctors once interpreted the human body through the lens of light — X-rays, MRIs, tissue samples. Now they interpret it through the lens of algorithms. But as these models grow more complex, the physician's role risks shifting from interpreter of the patient to interpreter of the machine's interpretation. The distance between illness and understanding grows — a semantic cave illuminated by computation.

We believe we have escaped ignorance by illuminating the world with data. Yet, in doing so, we may have entered a new kind of cave — one *brilliantly lit but existentially detached.* The walls now shimmer with infinite information, but the essence — the human meaning of health and disease — still lies beyond reach. The light that once symbolized enlightenment now blinds us with overexposure.

In this paradoxical illumination, AI has become both our guide and our new chain. It releases us from error but binds us to dependency. We no longer see the world directly; we see the world through the machine's geometry.

So the question remains — one that philosophy must now ask medicine:

Is knowledge illuminated by algorithms or obscured by them?

If Plato's cave was a metaphor for the limits of perception, the Cave of Data is a warning about the limits of computation. The walls are brighter, the shadows sharper, but the mystery remains. Truth has not disappeared — it has simply moved deeper into the code.

Reflection – Intelligence Without Awareness

Artificial intelligence now performs what was once considered a uniquely human act — it *knows.* It identifies, predicts, and reasons in ways that appear indistinguishable from cognition. Yet beneath its extraordinary performance lies a silent void — an intelligence without awareness. The machine knows, but it does not *know that it knows.* It sees, but it never *sees itself seeing.*

This distinction — subtle yet absolute — separates artificial cognition from human consciousness. When a human perceives, perception loops back into the self. The doctor who observes a scan is not only interpreting what is seen but also *experiencing the act of interpretation.* Awareness becomes a feedback circuit — perception informs identity, and identity shapes perception. We don't just process data; we locate ourselves within it. A physician doesn't merely recognize a tumor; they feel its implication — the weight of responsibility, the empathy for the patient, the humility before uncertainty. Seeing, for us, is always entangled with being.

AI, in contrast, operates in a pure, detached flow. It performs perception as function, not as experience. It lacks the recursive dimension that turns knowledge into understanding. The Digital Eye can process a million images and generate flawless classifications, but it remains blind to its own blindness. It cannot question the meaning of its perception because meaning, to it, does not exist — only data correlations do. Its awareness does not awaken; it only executes.

This absence of self-reference produces a paradoxical kind of perfection. The AI never hesitates, never doubts, never feels the tremor of uncertainty that defines human inquiry. But that same flawlessness is also its limitation. Without the humility of *not knowing*, there is no curiosity, and without curiosity, there can be no discovery. Every great leap in human knowledge — from Newton's gravity to Curie's radioactivity — began not with certainty, but with a question. The machine, in its current form, cannot question; it can only calculate.

Here lies the hidden cost of machine intelligence: it is precise but incapable of wisdom. Wisdom, after all, is born from reflection

— the fusion of knowledge with awareness of its limits. The AI does not reflect; it reproduces. It learns patterns, but it cannot examine purpose. It improves accuracy, but it cannot contemplate consequence.

Therefore, as we welcome these tireless observers into the clinic, a new ethical structure becomes necessary — one where human oversight serves as the conscience of artificial intelligence. The physician's judgment, empathy, and doubt must remain as the moral feedback loop that AI cannot form on its own. Machines can extend perception, but humans must still define meaning. The algorithm may flag a shadow; the doctor must decide what the shadow *means*.

AI's intelligence, in its brilliance, reminds us of something deeply humbling: our own dependence on awareness for meaning. In teaching machines to see, we have learned that vision itself is not the miracle — consciousness is.

"The machine sees everything but understands nothing — and still, it teaches us how little we know about seeing."

This is perhaps the most profound irony of the digital age — that in creating intelligence without awareness, humanity has come face to face with the limits of its own understanding. The machine's blindness to meaning mirrors our own blindness to being. Its silence is a reflection — not of ignorance, but of perfection stripped of purpose. And in that silence, we are reminded that to truly know, one must also *feel.*

Diagnosis Without a Doctor

The Digital Eye has learned to see — not just to observe, but to discern. It has mastered perception with mechanical grace, free from distraction, emotion, or fatigue. Yet sight, no matter how perfect, was never the end goal. In medicine, to *see* is only the beginning; to *decide* is the essence. And that is precisely where the next evolution begins.

As artificial intelligence grows confident in its perception, it inevitably begins to act. Once designed to assist, it now begins to infer, recommend, and predict — crossing the threshold from observation to decision. The system that once whispered suggestions into a clinician's ear now quietly drafts full reports, complete with diagnostic impressions and probable treatment paths. In many hospitals, these AI-generated insights are so accurate that doctors rarely disagree. The machine no longer asks to participate; it simply performs.

This marks a profound philosophical shift in medicine — from *seeing* to *deciding*, from *assisting* to *autonomy*. It is one thing for a machine to process an image; it is quite another for it to define what that image *means*. When the algorithm identifies pneumonia or early-stage cancer, it is not simply reading data; it is shaping destiny. Every diagnosis is an act of authority, and authority without awareness is power without conscience.

The ethical question now emerges with new urgency: if AI can diagnose better than most doctors, should it be allowed to? And if it is, who bears the moral weight of its conclusions? The developer? The hospital? The silent observer who approved its use? Medicine, once the art of human judgment, now finds itself negotiating with an intelligence that neither judges nor doubts.

This transition is not merely technological — it is existential. We are entering an era where decisions are made without deliberation, where responsibility may dissolve into the algorithmic fog of collective approval. The doctor remains in the room, but increasingly as a validator, not a visionary.

In the next chapter, we step into this uncharted territory — where machines diagnose with certainty and humans struggle with consequence. We will explore real-world deployments where *Doctor AI* has already begun issuing clinical verdicts, and we will confront the philosophical tension between trust and abdication.

For the moment, it is enough to acknowledge that the digital gaze no longer stops at seeing. It moves — silently, inevitably — toward decision.

"Having learned to see without eyes, the machine now dares to diagnose without permission."

Chapter 3 – Diagnosis Without a Doctor

When the machine speaks, who listens—and who is responsible?

The emergency room was chaos — flashing monitors, the rhythm of urgency. Amid the noise, one screen remained eerily calm. A CT scan appeared, and before the attending physician could adjust the contrast, a soft alert glowed on the corner: *"Intracranial hemorrhage detected – probability 0.97."*

No one had asked the machine for an opinion. It had spoken on its own.

The radiologist confirmed the finding within minutes — the AI was right. But as relief swept through the team, a quiet realization followed: the diagnosis had already been made before any human had looked. The authority of medicine had shifted, almost imperceptibly, from the physician's judgment to the algorithm's confidence.

In that moment, a new question entered the clinic — not whether machines *can* diagnose, but whether humans still *need* to.

The First Autonomous Diagnosis

The night shift at the hospital had settled into its familiar rhythm — the hum of fluorescent lights, the muted chatter of nurses, the low pulse of machines watching over the living. In the emergency imaging suite, the radiologist hadn't yet arrived at his console when a soft chime broke the monotony. On the monitor, a line of text appeared in calm, neutral font:

"Intracranial hemorrhage detected – probability: 0.97."

The machine had seen what no human eye had yet observed. By the time the radiologist logged in, the analysis was complete. The CT scan displayed a glowing red outline around the bleed, coordinates marked, measurements taken, urgency classified. The doctor scrolled through the slices, verifying out of habit — and yes, it was correct. The patient was prepped for surgery within minutes, the system's alert already integrated into the clinical workflow.

Everyone moved on. No one paused to consider the implication. Yet something irreversible had occurred: the *first diagnosis* that required no doctor. The machine had not only assisted — it had *acted.* It had interpreted, decided, and announced a finding before any human had participated in the process.

The radiologist later described the moment as both astonishing and disquieting. "It was right," he said, "but I didn't make the call." It was not fear he felt, but displacement — a subtle awareness that the locus of authority had shifted. The act of diagnosis, once a deeply human synthesis of observation and judgment, had been reduced to an algorithmic inference. The physician's role had quietly changed from *discoverer* to *confirmer.*

What was once assistive intelligence had evolved into autonomous inference — a system that doesn't merely suggest but concludes. The human presence, while still necessary, now serves as validation, not origin. Oversight remains, but increasingly as ritual — the comforting illusion of control in a process already decided by computation.

This moment marks the true threshold of modern medicine's transformation. For the first time, *decision precedes deliberation.* The diagnosis is not derived from thought; it is generated from pattern.

The machine does not reason; it recognizes. And yet, its recognition carries consequence — life, death, treatment, cost.

Here lies the philosophical tremor beneath the technological triumph:

Can correctness exist without conscience?

When a machine is right, it is *mathematically* right — but not *morally* right. It cannot feel relief at being correct or guilt at being wrong. Its intelligence lacks the weight of awareness, the humility of uncertainty, the empathy that gives medicine its soul. It may save a life, but it cannot value it.

And so, the emergency room that night became more than a scene of clinical efficiency; it became a quiet parable for the future of healing. The light on the monitor was not just an alert — it was a signal from the next era of medicine: a world where seeing has evolved into deciding, and where perfection may no longer require participation.

The New Clinical Frontier – Real-World Deployments and Accuracy Metrics

The era of speculation has quietly given way to deployment. The age of "experimental" medical AI is over; the *clinical frontier* is already here. What once existed only in research labs and glossy tech presentations now operates silently across hospitals, clinics, and even smartphones — diagnosing, triaging, and predicting, often before a human ever intervenes.

Across the world, a new class of autonomous and semi-autonomous diagnostic systems has begun reshaping how medicine works — and, perhaps more profoundly, how it *thinks*.

Aidoc and Zebra Medical Vision – The Eyes That Never Blink

These platforms represent the practical face of radiological AI. In emergency departments from Tel Aviv to New York, Aidoc scans CT and MRI images in real time, identifying intracranial hemorrhages, pulmonary embolisms, and fractures. Its alerts appear on radiologists' dashboards within seconds, often before the first manual read begins. Similarly, Zebra Medical Vision processes millions of anonymized scans to detect early signs of cardiovascular and skeletal disorders, providing triage prioritization that saves precious minutes — minutes that, in trauma care, often mean survival.

Clinical audits reveal that such systems consistently achieve sensitivity and specificity above 90%, outperforming fatigued human observers during long shifts. Yet, radiologists rarely describe these tools as replacements; they call them *co-workers*. The difference is subtle but essential: machines deliver precision, humans deliver meaning.

IDx-DR and Google's ARDA – The Eye That Diagnoses Itself

In 2018, IDx-DR became the first AI system to receive FDA approval for fully autonomous diagnosis — no physician oversight required. Designed to detect diabetic retinopathy, the system captures retinal images and independently determines whether a patient should be referred to an ophthalmologist. Its accuracy exceeded 87% sensitivity and 90% specificity in trials, rivaling expert graders.

Google's ARDA (Automated Retinal Disease Assessment) expanded this vision to global scale, integrating AI-based retinal screening in countries like Thailand and India, where ophthalmologists are scarce. The result: thousands of patients screened within hours, something no human workforce could achieve.

Yet here lies the quiet unease — the patients' diagnoses now arrive without a human name attached. The act of interpretation, once profoundly relational, has become infrastructural.

PathAI – Reading the Invisible City of Cells

In pathology, PathAI revolutionized how biopsy slides are analyzed. Whole-slide images, each comprising billions of pixels, are fed into deep-learning systems capable of identifying malignancies with uncanny precision. These models achieve AUC scores above 0.95, meaning their performance closely matches or even surpasses the world's best pathologists.

The advantage lies not in insight but in endurance: the machine can review thousands of slides without error, fatigue, or emotional influence. Still, many pathologists describe a strange loss — the erosion of the tactile relationship between the microscope and the mind. The digital glass may be cleaner, but the human gaze feels displaced.

CardioSignal, AliveCor, and Eko – The Heart in Code

In cardiology, AI now listens as attentively as any physician.

- CardioSignal detects early signs of heart failure by analyzing micro-vibrations through smartphone sensors.
- AliveCor's KardiaMobile records electrocardiograms on consumer devices, diagnosing atrial fibrillation within seconds.
- Eko merges digital stethoscopes with deep-learning algorithms to detect murmurs and arrhythmias at the point

of care.

Each tool extends medicine's reach beyond hospitals into homes, making continuous self-diagnosis possible — and continuous dependence inevitable.

Performance by the Numbers – Accuracy Without Awareness

The statistical story is impressive. Across multiple modalities — radiology, ophthalmology, pathology, and cardiology — AI systems routinely demonstrate:

- Sensitivity and specificity above 90%, sometimes exceeding expert consensus.
- Area Under the Curve (AUC) values surpassing 0.95, representing near-perfect discrimination between healthy and diseased states.
- Consistency far superior to humans, eliminating the variability caused by fatigue, mood, or bias.

Where doctors disagree, AI remains stable. Where humans hesitate, AI commits. And where human intuition falters, AI's pattern recognition holds steady.

Yet the paradox endures: machines outperform humans statistically but underperform them ethically. The algorithm never forgets, never doubts — but also never empathizes, never questions the consequences of being right.

Case Reflection – The Silent Hero in the Emergency Room

In countless hospitals worldwide, AI-driven triage systems already detect life-threatening conditions *minutes* before human review. A pulmonary embolism flagged early in a CT scan saves a life; a stroke caught faster prevents paralysis. These events unfold daily, quietly, without ceremony.

And yet, when success is recorded, the acknowledgment still goes to the physician who confirmed the finding — not to the code that first saw it. Doctors hesitate to credit the machine fully, perhaps out of professional caution, perhaps out of instinctive preservation of identity. For to admit that the machine *diagnosed first* is to concede that the hierarchy of knowledge has changed.

The new clinical frontier is not defined by technology alone, but by psychology — by how humanity negotiates partnership with precision. AI has already proven that it can diagnose faster and more consistently. What remains uncertain is whether we, as a species, can adapt to a world where *knowing* precedes *understanding.*

The hospital of tomorrow may be filled with algorithms that see perfectly — but it will still need humans who know *why seeing matters.*

Regulation of Machine Authority – FDA Approvals and Global Adoption

As artificial intelligence crossed the threshold from experiment to clinical implementation, it entered a domain once reserved for physicians, hospitals, and legal systems — the domain of *authority.* The machine's competence is no longer in question; its legitimacy is. Medicine, once governed by licenses, credentials, and ethics, now faces a new challenge: how to regulate an entity that performs like a doctor, but isn't human enough to be held accountable.

The regulatory world, unprepared for this transformation, had to invent a new category — "Software as a Medical Device (SaMD)." Under this definition, an algorithm itself becomes a medical instrument, capable of diagnosis, prognosis, or therapeutic decision-making. This shift from *tool* to *actor* marks one of the most significant legal reclassifications in modern healthcare. What was once "decision-support software" — a digital assistant to help doctors — is now, in certain contexts, an independent decision-maker.

Milestone 1: The FDA Approval of IDx-DR (2018)

The turning point came in 2018 when the U.S. Food and Drug Administration (FDA) approved IDx-DR, the first autonomous AI diagnostic system that required no physician involvement. Designed to detect diabetic retinopathy from retinal images, it was the first machine authorized to make a medical decision *on its own.* The FDA's reasoning was pragmatic: the system had demonstrated sensitivity and specificity equal to or exceeding human experts in clinical trials. For rural or under-resourced clinics with no ophthalmologist on-site, it provided an accessible and reliable screening solution.

This single approval symbolized the moment medicine officially recognized non-human intelligence as diagnostically competent. The machine had earned not just performance credibility, but *legal authority.*

Milestone 2: CE and CDSCO Approvals for Radiology Algorithms

Following the FDA, the European Union (EU) introduced its own standards under the CE marking framework, requiring rigorous documentation of algorithmic validation, bias control, and post-deployment monitoring. Systems like Aidoc, Lunit, and Zebra Medical Vision received CE certification for radiology triage, allowing clinical use across multiple European nations.

Meanwhile, in India, the Central Drugs Standard Control Organization (CDSCO) began granting limited clearances to AI systems used for tuberculosis screening and radiology assistance under the Digital Health Mission. The adoption was notably pragmatic — driven less by regulatory perfection and more by healthcare necessity. For nations with large populations and few specialists, autonomy became not a luxury, but a lifeline.

Milestone 3: WHO's Ethical Framework (2021)

By 2021, the World Health Organization released a comprehensive framework for Ethics and Governance of AI for Health — a global attempt to unify standards around transparency, safety, accountability, and inclusivity. The report emphasized six guiding principles: human autonomy, well-being, safety, transparency, accountability, and sustainability. It warned that while AI may enhance equity, it could just as easily amplify inequality if deployed without oversight. The WHO did not regulate — it reminded the world that regulation without comprehension is illusion.

Global Contrasts – Three Modes of Adoption

- **The United States:** Prioritizes *commercial integration.* Regulation evolves reactively — innovation first, ethics later. The FDA often relies on *real-world performance data* rather than pre-approval clarity. The result is a fast-moving market with frequent post-approval corrections. The American model celebrates disruption but risks ethical turbulence.
- **The European Union:** Adopts *precautionary rigor.* Its regulatory bodies treat algorithms as potential medical liabilities from the start. Strict data-protection laws (GDPR) and AI Act proposals enforce explainability and fairness. Progress is slower, but trust runs deeper.

- **Asia (India, China, Singapore):** Exhibits *grassroots pragmatism.* Adoption is driven by accessibility and public-health scale. AI tools are deployed rapidly in rural clinics, mobile apps, and telemedicine networks. Regulation often follows innovation — a reflection of societal urgency over bureaucratic restraint.

Each approach reveals a different cultural philosophy of technology: the U.S. trusts performance, Europe trusts process, and Asia trusts potential.

Philosophical Undercurrent – The Law's Blind Spot

The law, designed for human accountability, struggles to regulate what it cannot comprehend. When intelligence lacks intent, can it possess guilt? When an algorithm makes a correct diagnosis, who deserves credit — the coder, the clinician, or the machine itself? And when it errs, who bears responsibility for the harm — the operator who trusted it or the architecture that learned without malice?

In conventional ethics, *responsibility* is a consequence of *awareness.* But AI operates without awareness, and yet its consequences are profoundly real. This disconnect between power and personhood leaves regulation in a gray zone.

The machine acts like a doctor but cannot be punished like one. It commits no crime, but its precision can still cause pain.

Ethical Reflection – Shared Authority, Divided Accountability

Modern healthcare now operates within a web of shared responsibility — a triad of code, clinician, and corporation. The doctor deploys the AI, the developer designs it, and the hospital implements it. Each claims partial ownership of success and partial distance from failure.

The result is a strange new hierarchy of healing — where accountability diffuses as intelligence concentrates. A perfect system for progress, and a dangerous one for justice.

The regulation of machine authority is not merely a legal evolution; it is a moral reformation. For the first time, medicine must govern an intelligence that does not obey, apologize, or understand.

Philosophical question: *How does law protect humanity from what is not human, yet acts as if it were?*

As *Doctor AI* steps deeper into the clinic, the courtroom must evolve alongside it — or risk becoming another spectator in a theater where accountability dissolves into data.

Beyond the Hospital – Tele-Diagnostics and Rural Reach

The promise of *Doctor AI* is not confined to gleaming metropolitan hospitals or high-end research centers. Its true potential — and its greatest test — lies far from these institutions, in the dust and distance of the developing world, where doctors are scarce, equipment is outdated, and access to healthcare is often determined by geography rather than need.

In these remote corners, AI-powered tele-diagnostics have begun to perform a quiet revolution. With little more than a smartphone, a solar charger, and a mobile data signal, clinics that once struggled to provide basic care now conduct digital screenings once thought possible only in advanced hospitals.

Democratizing Diagnosis through Technology

AI-driven telemedicine platforms are rapidly reshaping access to diagnosis across continents.

- Smartphone-based retinal scanners, powered by algorithms derived from projects like IDx-DR and Google's ARDA, now screen for diabetic retinopathy and glaucoma in small clinics and even roadside camps. Health workers, not ophthalmologists, take the images; the AI interprets them within minutes. What once required a city hospital and a specialist now fits into a handheld lens attached to a mobile phone.
- Chest X-ray AI systems, such as those developed for tuberculosis (TB) detection by companies like Qure.ai and Zebra Medical Vision, are being deployed in India, Nigeria, and Kenya. These models scan portable X-rays for pulmonary lesions, flagging likely TB cases on the spot — a critical breakthrough in regions where delays often mean death.
- Handheld ultrasound devices equipped with embedded inference models — like Butterfly iQ and Philips Lumify — are redefining prenatal care, cardiac monitoring, and abdominal diagnostics. A nurse in a village can now capture images and have AI interpret them in real time, bypassing both specialist shortages and infrastructural constraints.

These technologies embody the dream of democratized diagnosis — the notion that quality healthcare should not depend on proximity to a city or a specialist.

Narrative Case – The Clinic in the Desert

In a small clinic on the edge of Rajasthan's Thar Desert, a young nurse adjusts her mobile phone on a tripod. The temperature outside hovers above forty degrees, but inside, a solar panel hums quietly, powering a portable X-ray machine. A middle-aged farmer, coughing for weeks, sits nervously as the scan is taken.

Within forty seconds, the mobile screen flashes: "TB Detected – High Probability (0.91). Immediate referral recommended." No radiologist, no lab technician — just an algorithm, trained on millions of images across the world, issuing a verdict in real time. The nurse uploads the result to the district health database. Within minutes, the patient is scheduled for confirmatory testing at the nearest hospital, forty kilometers away.

For the first time, diagnosis has arrived *before distance could deny it.* In that dusty room, the machine is not replacing the doctor — it is becoming the bridge to one.

The Triple Benefit: Accessibility, Affordability, Immediacy

1. **Accessibility:** AI bypasses physical limitations — no need for specialized infrastructure, expensive machines, or human expertise on site. A phone and a network connection are enough to summon expertise once confined to global capitals.
2. **Affordability:** The cost per diagnosis drops drastically. Once purchased or licensed, an AI model can process thousands of cases with negligible marginal cost, transforming healthcare economics for low-income regions.
3. **Immediacy:** Time, the most precious resource in emergency care, collapses. What once took days or weeks — transporting scans, waiting for doctors, retrieving results — now unfolds within minutes.

For communities historically excluded from medical infrastructure, AI is not just an innovation — it is emancipation.

But the Shadows Remain: Risks and Limitations

Beneath the optimism, the reality is uneven. Many rural networks operate on unstable internet connections; models trained on urban datasets may falter in different demographic or environmental contexts. Dust on a lens, poor lighting, or low-resolution imaging can distort results.

The absence of *clinical validation* and *professional supervision* means that some diagnoses go unverified. A false positive can send a poor farmer on a 100-kilometer journey; a false negative can seal his fate. AI, for all its efficiency, cannot substitute for the nuanced judgment that understands *how to act on error.*

Moreover, unmonitored deployment creates new ethical dilemmas. Who monitors the performance of these models in rural clinics? Who ensures updates, retraining, and recalibration? The developers? The governments? Or the communities themselves, who barely understand the system's logic but live with its consequences?

Reflection – Equality of Access, Inequality of Accuracy

AI has succeeded in delivering equality of access, but not yet equality of accuracy. A rural clinic may use the same algorithm as a global hospital, but not the same infrastructure, calibration, or human oversight. The technology is identical; the context is not.

The paradox is profound: in making healthcare *available* to everyone, we risk making it *reliable* for no one — unless we reimagine responsibility alongside reach.

Reflection: *AI has carried medicine to the farthest corners of the world, yet it still struggles to see clearly where light is scarce.*

The digital doctor has extended its hand to the forgotten — but it will take human wisdom, not machine vision, to ensure that the help it offers is truly healing.

The Rise of Self-Diagnosing Populations

The waiting room is vanishing. Across the world, millions of people now carry in their pockets what once filled hospitals: a pulse monitor, an ECG reader, a skin analyzer, a virtual clinician. Diagnosis, once mediated by the gatekeepers of medicine, has slipped quietly into the hands of the public. The question is no longer *"Can machines diagnose?"* — but *"Should everyone?"*

From Clinic to Pocket – The New Age of Consumer Diagnostics

A decade ago, medical technology was institutional — heavy, expensive, and restricted to trained professionals. Today, it has become personal, portable, and app-based. The line between *patient* and *practitioner* is dissolving.

- **AliveCor / KardiaMobile:** A small sensor that attaches to a smartphone, recording medical-grade electrocardiograms within seconds. It detects atrial fibrillation and other rhythm disorders with clinical accuracy, instantly advising whether to seek medical attention. Millions now check their hearts between meetings, on airplanes, or in bed — the cardiologist in the palm.
- **SkinVision and MoleScope:** AI-powered skin-cancer detection apps that photograph moles or lesions and return risk scores in minutes. They claim early detection saves lives; dermatologists warn that false alarms cause unnecessary anxiety. The phone becomes a mirror not of vanity but of mortality.
- **Ada Health, Babylon, WebMD AI:** Symptom-checker apps that invite users to describe their pain in words and sliders, returning differential diagnoses, probabilities, and

next steps. For many, they are the first doctor they consult — one who never sleeps, never judges, and never charges.

What these tools have achieved is extraordinary: they have democratized diagnosis, giving billions the ability to interpret their bodies through the logic of data. Yet what they have also created is a new psychological condition — the *illusion of certainty.*

Empowerment or Paranoia? The Psychology of Self-Diagnosis

The appeal of self-diagnosis is deeply emotional. It promises control in a world of medical opacity. The act of scanning one's heartbeat or skin spot feels empowering — a reclaiming of agency from institutions that often feel inaccessible or indifferent. Patients no longer wait for permission to know; they simply check.

But this empowerment carries an unseen shadow — algorithmic anxiety. Every vibration in the chest becomes a signal, every twinge a possible threat. A benign rash becomes a malignancy in waiting; a skipped heartbeat becomes an impending attack. The algorithm's cold precision often collides with the mind's fragile calm.

We are witnessing the birth of a new paradoxical species — *the anxious informed.* People who know more about their risk factors than ever before, yet feel less certain about their health.

Social Consequences – Medicine Without Doctors

As these tools spread, society itself begins to recalibrate around them. Pharmacies now sell diagnostic wearables. Insurance companies incentivize continuous self-monitoring. Employers gamify health tracking. The ecosystem of medicine is shifting from consultation to computation.

The subtle but profound consequence is this: *medical advice is being replaced by algorithmic reassurance or alarm.* Instead of a doctor's reasoned explanation, users receive binary verdicts — *"Normal"* or *"Abnormal."* The gray zone of uncertainty, once filled by conversation, is now filled by silence or panic. The ancient ritual of trust between patient and healer is being digitized — converted from empathy to probability.

In a world where every citizen can self-diagnose, the very meaning of expertise begins to blur. If everyone can detect a problem, who decides what counts as illness? If every device can quantify risk, who defines what it means to be well?

The Philosophical Inquiry – The Erosion of Expertise

Medicine, for centuries, has rested on a sacred asymmetry — the patient's vulnerability balanced by the doctor's wisdom. But as machines deliver diagnostic precision directly to the individual, this asymmetry collapses. Knowledge is no longer scarce; it is everywhere. Yet understanding remains as rare as ever.

The philosopher Ivan Illich once warned that industrial societies risk *"medicalizing life itself."* Today, AI has made that prophecy digital. Every heartbeat, every calorie, every fluctuation is now a potential data point of disorder. The boundary between living and being monitored has all but disappeared.

Philosophical question: *When everyone can diagnose, does expertise lose meaning—or does it finally become moral rather than technical?*

Perhaps the future doctor will not be the one who knows the most, but the one who can *interpret meaning* amid algorithmic noise — the curator of understanding in an age of abundance.

The Paradox of Modern Autonomy

This is the paradox of our time: we trust machines over doctors, yet we seek doctors to reassure us about machines. We ask AI if we are sick, then ask humans if the AI might be wrong. The authority we've transferred to technology we immediately retrieve for comfort.

This recursive loop defines the psychology of the digital patient — hyper-informed yet emotionally uncertain. We crave precision, but long for empathy. We want autonomy, but not isolation.

And so, the human role persists, not as a dispenser of knowledge, but as a *translator of meaning* — the only voice capable of turning information into reassurance.

Reflection: In teaching machines to diagnose us, we have learned that what we sought was never certainty — it was understanding. The machine gives us data; the doctor still gives us peace.

Automation and Ignorance – Does Technology Cure or Multiply It?

The central technophilosophical question of our time can be framed in one line:

"Does automation cure ignorance, or merely automate it?"

We created machines to overcome human limitations — to remove error, bias, and fatigue from judgment. Yet, in doing so, we may have built systems that remove *understanding* as well. The paradox is subtle but profound: as AI grows more intelligent, human knowledge becomes shallower. Automation corrects our mistakes, but also weakens the muscles that once learned from them.

When Accuracy Creates New Error

In medicine, AI's precision is undeniable. Machines have outperformed doctors in detecting lung nodules, skin lesions, retinal damage, and cardiac anomalies. They spot what humans miss — the microscopic, the statistical, the hidden. But while AI reduces *technical* error, it introduces a new category altogether: *interpretive* error.

Consider a patient using a skin-cancer detection app. The AI flags a mole as "suspicious – high probability." The patient, terrified, assumes malignancy and rushes into unnecessary biopsies and sleepless nights. In truth, the mole is benign; the algorithm's caution is statistical, not diagnostic. The machine was not wrong — it was misread. Here, ignorance hasn't been cured; it has been *mechanized.*

Automation doesn't remove human fallibility — it *relocates* it. The error shifts from perception to interpretation, from doctor to device, from misreading the body to misreading the machine.

The Comfort of Delegation – Cognitive Atrophy in the Digital Age

As AI grows more capable, humans grow more dependent. The modern doctor, aided by automated imaging tools and predictive analytics, often accepts the machine's verdict without full understanding of its logic. The patient, empowered by self-diagnostic apps, often stops questioning once the screen provides an answer.

This dependence mirrors what psychologists call the "Google Effect" — the phenomenon where easy access to information reduces our inclination to remember or reason. In medicine, it manifests as a quiet cognitive erosion: why memorize anatomy when the software highlights it? why interpret patterns when the algorithm labels them?

The very success of automation risks producing a generation of clinicians and patients who no longer *think diagnostically,* but *consume diagnoses.* The mind grows passive when certainty becomes a service.

In this sense, automation may not be curing ignorance — it may be outsourcing it.

Democratization or Dependence – Who Controls the Cure?

AI has undoubtedly democratized access to medical knowledge. Millions now possess diagnostic tools once reserved for institutions. Yet, beneath this surface of empowerment lies an invisible consolidation of control.

Every self-diagnostic app, every AI-driven medical platform, runs on datasets owned by corporations or governments. The more individuals use these systems, the more data they generate — data that flows upward, not outward. In effect, AI decentralizes access but centralizes authority.

Medicine, once a dialogue between doctor and patient, risks becoming a transaction between user and algorithm — mediated by entities that neither heal nor answer. The patient gains information but loses autonomy over its interpretation. The algorithm knows more about the user than the user knows about the algorithm.

Thus, while automation distributes knowledge, it simultaneously concentrates power.

Example – The Misread Machine

A case from Singapore illustrates this paradox vividly. A patient using an AI-powered cardiac health app received an alert reading *"possible arrhythmia detected."* Alarmed, he visited three specialists, underwent multiple tests, and endured weeks of anxiety — only to discover that his smartwatch had misinterpreted motion artifacts from exercise as cardiac irregularities.

The AI wasn't at fault — it performed its task faithfully. The misunderstanding lay in the *human expectation* that precision equals truth. In seeking certainty, the patient found confusion. The technology eliminated ignorance about heart rhythm, but multiplied ignorance about *meaning*.

Insight – The Paradox of Automated Understanding

Automation, by design, simplifies complexity. It turns uncertainty into clarity, probabilities into answers. Yet, in doing so, it often erases the space where thinking happens — the very uncertainty that once forced humans to inquire, reason, and learn.

Insight: *In curing uncertainty, AI may be multiplying misunderstanding.*

The machine replaces not just our errors, but our process of discovery. And when discovery is automated, comprehension quietly disappears.

We are entering a future where ignorance will not look like absence of knowledge — it will look like the presence of unquestioned information. Automation will not make us less ignorant by giving us more answers; it will make us *differently ignorant* by removing the need to ask.

And so, the ultimate task for *Doctor AI* — and for humanity — is not to automate certainty, but to preserve wonder: the willingness to doubt, to reflect, and to seek meaning in what even machines claim to know.

Reflection – The Disappearing Physician

The doctor still stands in the room — the white coat remains, the stethoscope still hangs — but something fundamental has changed.

The authority that once radiated from the physician's presence has migrated into the glowing interface beside them. The monitor speaks first. The human confirms.

The physician's role, once defined by discovery and discernment, is slowly being rewritten as verification. Where doctors once searched, they now *supervise.* Where they once questioned, they now *confirm.* In the age of algorithmic medicine, the clinician has become less the diagnostician and more the algorithmic editor — checking the machine's output for errors rather than exploring the unknown. The joy of finding a hidden truth in a sea of uncertainty — once the essence of medicine's artistry — is being replaced by the mechanical comfort of correctness.

From Diagnostician to Interpreter of Code

The doctor of the twentieth century relied on intuition honed by experience — the subtle pattern recognition born of decades of listening, touching, and observing. The doctor of the twenty-first century relies increasingly on pattern recognition *outsourced* to machines. The clinical gaze, once human and subjective, is now mediated through statistical certainty.

The modern physician interprets machine verdicts more than human symptoms. They read not faces but probability maps, not pulse rhythms but confidence intervals. The patient becomes a dataset; the diagnosis, a decimal.

And though the results may be more precise, something irreplaceable is lost — the *interpretive intimacy* that made medicine a dialogue rather than a report.

The Emotional Cost of Detachment

When the act of diagnosis becomes automated, the doctor's emotional connection to the process — and to the patient — begins to thin. A clinician who once spent minutes listening to a patient's description of pain now glances at an AI-generated summary: "Possible early neuropathy. Recommend blood work." The conversation shortens. The trust weakens. The healing slows.

Patients, too, feel the change. The reassurance that once came from a doctor's eyes is now replaced by the sterile confidence of a screen. Even when the diagnosis is correct, the *experience* of care feels colder. In this new system, efficiency increases, but empathy evaporates. The machine may never err, but it never *cares.*

Medicine risks drifting into an ethical no-man's-land — between the safety of automation and the humanity of imperfection.

The Erosion of Professional Identity

Doctors often describe their work as a blend of science and art — the precise balance between objective knowledge and subjective wisdom. But as automation grows, the scales tip heavily toward the scientific. The art fades.

Young doctors entering the profession today are trained not just in anatomy and physiology, but in algorithmic literacy. They learn to read not only lab reports, but neural networks. Their challenge is no longer to diagnose disease, but to interpret diagnostics. In this transition, medicine risks creating a generation of professionals who know *how to verify* but not *how to wonder.*

The physician's intellect remains valuable, but their imagination — the ability to think beyond data — risks atrophy.

Medicine Without Empathy, or Medicine Without Error?

The ultimate philosophical tension of this new era can be reduced to a painful question:

Do we want medicine without empathy, or medicine without error?

Machines promise precision but no compassion. Humans offer care but make mistakes. Perfection, it turns out, comes at the cost of presence. And presence — the act of being fully human with another human in suffering — was always medicine's greatest cure.

As the Digital Doctor rises, the human doctor must redefine their worth. It is no longer in detecting disease, but in *contextualizing* it. It is no longer in knowing more, but in feeling deeper. For when data becomes flawless, meaning must come from somewhere else — from the heart that still chooses to care.

"When knowledge becomes automatic, wisdom must become intentional."

Automation has conquered error; now humanity must conquer indifference. The doctor of the future may not hold the scalpel or the stethoscope — but they will hold something infinitely rarer: the courage to stay human when machines no longer need them.

In that fragile balance — between precision and presence, between knowing and understanding — lies the soul of medicine yet to be rediscovered.

The Human in the Loop

The rise of *Doctor AI* has taken us from sight to judgment, from data to decision, from human intuition to machine inference. The digital doctor now perceives, predicts, and pronounces. Yet in this new world of algorithmic medicine, one truth refuses to fade — the system, however perfect, still needs someone watching *it*.

After the euphoria of automation comes the sobering realization of *responsibility*. Machines may act faster, but they do not *intend.* They perform without awareness, diagnose without empathy, and succeed without accountability. It is here, at this intersection between performance and purpose, that the human role returns — not as operator, but as *moral equilibrium.*

As *Doctor AI* steps deeper into decision-making, the need for *human oversight* becomes not a safety measure but a moral necessity. The clinician's presence ensures that efficiency does not silence ethics, that precision does not outgrow compassion. The new physician's task is not to compete with the algorithm, but to *align* with it — to interpret, to restrain, and to remind.

The next chapter, *"The Human in the Loop,"* explores this delicate reintroduction of control — the architecture of partnership where machines calculate but humans *care.* It will examine how oversight, feedback, and ethical reasoning can transform automation from a mechanical force into a moral collaborator. It will question not how to outsmart the algorithm, but how to infuse it with *conscience.*

This is the new Hippocratic frontier: to ensure that technological perfection does not come at the cost of human purpose. The physician's role evolves, but it does not disappear; it deepens.

"The doctor has not vanished; he now watches the watcher — ensuring that perfection remembers to care."

Chapter 4 – The Human in the Loop

Perfection needs purpose; precision needs conscience.

The scan was flawless. Every pixel analyzed, every anomaly measured. The algorithm had already declared its verdict — *benign.* Yet the radiologist lingered. Something about the contour felt wrong, not statistically, but instinctively. He overrode the AI, ordered a biopsy, and days later the results confirmed malignancy. The machine had missed what the mind had felt.

In that brief act of hesitation, the doctor reappeared — not as a technician, but as a conscience.

This is the paradox of modern medicine: machines may deliver precision, but only humans can deliver *purpose.* The loop is closing between intelligence and intuition, yet the future of healing depends not on which sees better, but on which remembers *why* we see at all.

Watching the Watcher

The radiologist stared at the monitor, his finger hovering over the trackpad. On the screen, the algorithm's neat annotation glowed in amber: "Possible tumor detected – probability: 0.89."

The lesion was faint, almost indistinguishable — a smudge on an otherwise clean image. Years of training told him it was nothing, perhaps an artifact, perhaps a shadow of motion. Yet the AI's confidence was unnervingly high. The system had processed a million such scans, learned from thousands of confirmed cases, and now presented its verdict with mathematical composure.

He zoomed in. Zoomed out. Adjusted the contrast. Still unsure. In that moment, he realized the uncomfortable inversion of authority — the *machine* was now the confident one. He, the expert, was the skeptic.

The decision was his to make, but the *certainty* was no longer his to hold.

The New Tension: Who Is Right?

The modern clinic has become a stage for a new kind of epistemic tension — the silent debate between human judgment and algorithmic probability. Who is right — the doctor guided by intuition, or the machine armed with statistics?

The human mind works with experience, patterns, and context. It senses subtle asymmetries, interprets emotional cues, and weighs the meaning of consequence. But it also tires, doubts, and forgets. The machine, by contrast, never wavers, never hesitates, and never questions. It computes endlessly — detached, perfect, and blind.

For the first time in the history of medicine, knowledge has divided into two species: one that feels truth and one that calculates it. The physician must now navigate between them, caught between instinct and inference.

Every disagreement between doctor and machine is no longer just a diagnostic uncertainty; it is a philosophical duel — between confidence born of conscience and confidence born of computation.

The New Role: From Creator to Custodian

A generation ago, doctors were the *creators* of medical truth. They discovered diseases, identified patterns, and defined the standards by which health was measured. Their observations became the knowledge that machines would later learn from.

Today, that hierarchy has shifted. Doctors are no longer the authors of knowledge; they are its custodians. Their task is to verify, interpret, and validate what algorithms produce — to watch the watcher. The AI generates the insight; the human approves its reality. This new partnership transforms the doctor from explorer to editor, from diagnostician to arbiter of truth.

This redefined role is not a demotion of intellect, but a re-centering of ethics. The machine may predict outcomes, but only the human can assign them *meaning.*

Philosophical Prompt: The Weight of Awareness

This quiet scene — one scan, one probability, one hesitation — encapsulates the new moral architecture of medicine. The machine's intelligence is mechanical, its awareness nonexistent. It can detect, but it cannot *decide*. It can conclude, but it cannot *care.*

And so, the burden returns to the physician — not to outsmart the machine, but to uphold what the machine cannot feel: responsibility.

Philosophical prompt: *When intelligence becomes mechanical, responsibility must remain human.*

No matter how perfect the algorithm, the conscience of medicine cannot be outsourced. For while machines may process uncertainty with precision, only humans can bear its weight.

In the age of artificial diagnosis, the doctor's truest skill may no longer be in detecting illness — but in discerning when to trust what has already been detected.

The Validator's Burden – Redefining the Role of Clinicians

In the age of *Doctor AI,* the physician's desk has turned into a reviewing station. The scans arrive pre-analyzed, the lab reports pre-interpreted, and the algorithm's verdict — bold and color-coded — stares back from the screen before the clinician has even taken a breath. The rhythm of medical reasoning has changed. Once, the doctor pieced together fragments of uncertainty into a coherent diagnosis. Now, the coherence arrives first; the doctor's task is to confirm it.

A quiet but profound inversion has taken place in medicine's epistemic hierarchy: *the machine generates, and the human validates.*

From Discovery to Curation

Medicine has long been a field of discovery — of observation, correlation, and revelation. Each diagnosis was an act of synthesis, a marriage of science and intuition. The physician's authority rested on the ability to *see what others missed,* to assemble patterns into meaning through experience and empathy.

But as AI systems entered the diagnostic chain, this creative process began to shift. Algorithms now perform the synthesis, correlating billions of data points to predict outcomes that no human could compute. Doctors no longer discover patterns; they *curate* them. Their expertise is redirected from finding truth to verifying it.

The clinician becomes a custodian of algorithmic accuracy — the final checkpoint before the machine's knowledge turns into human consequence. In theory, this validation preserves safety; in practice, it redefines purpose.

The Physician as Validator

In this new order, physicians function as "validators" — a role both indispensable and paradoxically diminished. They must approve machine-derived conclusions, but often lack full visibility into how those conclusions were reached. The AI presents probability scores and visual heatmaps, but its reasoning remains abstract, buried in layers of neural logic.

Thus, doctors find themselves endorsing what they cannot fully explain — a tension that undercuts both confidence and control. Their signature on the report carries the moral and legal responsibility, even though the intellectual authorship belongs to the algorithm.

This inversion creates a subtle form of dependency. Doctors rely on machines not for efficiency, but for *assurance.* And yet, this assurance comes with an uneasy truth: validation may preserve safety, but it slowly erodes sovereignty.

Practical Implications – The Workflow of Trust

The new workflow of AI-assisted medicine mirrors the structure of aviation:

- The **algorithm** scans vast data streams, identifies anomalies, and issues alerts.
- The **clinician** reviews these alerts, compares them with clinical history, and either accepts or overrides the output.
- The **system** logs every decision, learning from both agreement and dissent.

Over time, this creates *diagnostic verification loops* — recursive cycles where the AI improves by observing human feedback, and humans adapt by observing AI consistency. The result is a dynamic of co-dependence: the system needs human judgment to evolve; the human needs machine validation to feel secure.

But this loop has a cost. Doctors begin to *self-correct* less, relying instead on algorithmic guidance. Clinical autonomy — once defined by independent reasoning — becomes procedural. Decision-making transforms into a review process. Medicine, once driven by the art of judgment, turns into an act of *approval.*

The Emotional Dimension – The Quiet Erosion of Confidence

For many physicians, the shift is not only procedural but deeply personal. The satisfaction of diagnostic insight — the thrill of discovery, the intuition confirmed — fades when the conclusion is pre-written. The mental rigor of uncertainty, once the crucible of medical growth, is replaced by algorithmic certainty.

This creates a new emotional strain: moral fatigue. Doctors find themselves torn between duty and doubt — compelled to validate a machine that rarely errs, yet aware that blind acceptance feels ethically hollow. Some confess to a strange loss of purpose: *"I save more lives, but I feel less like a doctor."*

The erosion of uncertainty has not brought peace; it has brought restlessness. The human mind, evolved to reason, now merely reviews. And in that quiet surrender of curiosity lies the slow disintegration of professional identity.

Insight – Validation Preserves Safety, but Erodes Identity

The validator's burden is paradoxical. It safeguards the system from catastrophic error — yet in doing so, it slowly strips the physician of the very thing that defined their calling: the right to *interpret reality through judgment, not just through compliance.*

Insight: *Validation may preserve safety, but it erodes identity — a new kind of moral fatigue.*

In the hospital of the future, the doctor may make fewer mistakes, but also fewer discoveries. And while the machine's precision may perfect the science of medicine, it is up to the human to preserve its art.

Trust, Liability, and Interpretability

In the age of algorithmic medicine, the heartbeat of trust no longer lies in the stethoscope — it pulses in the server. Yet the doctor who depends on the machine knows that trust in technology is never as clean as its code. It is built on performance, but eroded by opacity.

AI may predict disease more accurately than any radiologist alive, but when its logic remains invisible, the human who must act on its judgment stands on uncertain ground. The doctor trusts the output but fears the *reasoning.*

Trust – The Fragile Contract Between Human and Machine

Trust in medicine has always been intimate — built through conversation, empathy, and consistency. But algorithms cannot offer reassurance; they only deliver results. The trust between doctor and AI is, therefore, a strange and asymmetrical one: the machine is consistent, but not comprehensible.

Early studies reveal the paradox vividly. Physicians report higher *confidence* in AI's accuracy, yet lower *comfort* in its decisions. The very perfection that inspires admiration also breeds unease. They trust what it *does*, but not what it *means.*

This unease is not technical — it is philosophical. A doctor can explain her own decision, even if wrong; she cannot explain an algorithm's, even if right. Thus, trust becomes performative — based on track record, not understanding. It's faith, not knowledge.

The AI never lies, but it never explains.

Liability – When the Machine Is Wrong

The machine's precision may save countless lives, but what happens when it fails? When the algorithm misses a malignancy, misreads a scan, or produces a false negative that costs a life — who is responsible?

- The developer, who designed the algorithm?
- The hospital, which implemented it?
- Or the doctor, who approved the report bearing its conclusions?

The answer varies by jurisdiction, but the ambiguity remains global. Doctors find themselves in a new kind of legal limbo — bearing the ethical weight of decisions partially made by systems they neither wrote nor fully understand.

Case Reflections – The Shared Blame

- In 2022, a U.S. radiology clinic faced litigation after an AI-assisted tool failed to flag a lung nodule that later proved cancerous. The manufacturer denied fault, citing that the AI was "advisory." The radiologist claimed overreliance on hospital-mandated software. The court ruled neither side fully liable, introducing the term "shared responsibility" — a verdict that satisfied no one.
- In the EU, similar cases prompted the drafting of the AI Liability Directive, complementing the EU AI Act, which demands transparency, human oversight, and traceable logs for all "high-risk" medical algorithms.

- The FDA (U.S.) now classifies such systems as *Software as a Medical Device (SaMD)*, requiring documented risk assessment and physician accountability for final decisions.
- The WHO's 2021 Guidance on Ethics and Governance of AI in Health went further — demanding "explainability proportional to risk," a phrase both moral and impossible.

The law is trying to regulate something it cannot yet define: a decision made by non-human intelligence.

Interpretability – The Quest to Understand the Unseeable

To bridge this gap between faith and fear, researchers turned to Explainable AI (XAI) — systems designed to make black boxes translucent. These models attempt to show *why* an algorithm made a decision, using visualizations like saliency maps, Grad-CAM overlays, attention heatmaps, or feature-importance plots.

In radiology, this means the AI can highlight the precise pixels or patterns that influenced its classification — giving the doctor a sense of transparency. But the catch is profound: explanation does not equal understanding.

A colored heatmap does not reveal logic; it merely gestures at correlation. The doctor sees where the AI "looked," but not *how it thought.* True interpretability remains elusive, because the reasoning process of deep networks is not narrative — it is mathematical abstraction.

Thus, even the most "explainable" systems are, at best, mirrors showing shadows of their own cognition.

Interpretability comforts the conscience, but it does not illuminate the mind.

The Ethical Paradox – Transparency vs. Performance

This tension reaches its philosophical climax in the trade-off that defines the future of AI in healthcare:

- **Transparent AI** (simpler, explainable) is slower and less powerful — safe but limited.
- **Opaque AI** (deep, complex) is faster and more accurate — potent but unaccountable.

Every healthcare institution now faces this moral calculus: Do we prefer truth we can explain, or accuracy we can't?

The choice is no longer about technology — it is about values. Transparency satisfies ethics but may sacrifice outcomes. Opacity saves lives but undermines accountability. The former comforts humanity; the latter challenges it.

Reflection – The Anatomy of Trust

Trust in the age of *Doctor AI* is no longer about believing in people, but about believing in systems we cannot fully see. The doctor remains the visible face of invisible reasoning — signing off on diagnoses authored by code, shouldering accountability for knowledge that is no longer personal.

Philosophical Insight: *We built machines we could trust, but not question; and in doing so, we traded comprehension for certainty.*

In this new order, the doctor's task is not to rival the algorithm, but to guard the fragile balance between blind faith and moral doubt — to remind a world of flawless predictions that medicine without understanding is not yet healing.

When AI and Doctor Disagree – The Epistemic Conflict

The MRI image is clear. The algorithm has marked an irregular region in bright red — *"Possible early-stage glioma, 0.84 probability."* The radiologist disagrees. "Artifact," she says, "the contrast is off." She dismisses the flag, notes "no significant abnormality," and moves on.

Weeks later, the patient returns with worsening symptoms. A follow-up scan confirms the AI was right. The tumor had been there — faint, early, invisible to the human eye but legible to the machine's pattern.

A similar scene unfolds elsewhere: a pathologist examines a digital slide and questions the AI's assessment of "precancerous dysplasia." Months later, pathology consensus validates the algorithm's initial reading. The pattern that once looked like noise had meaning after all.

These are not stories of human failure; they are the signs of a new epistemic tension — the confrontation between two distinct ways of knowing.

The Epistemic Conflict – Two Intelligences, One Reality

Medicine has entered an era where truth is no longer singular. When a machine and a doctor look at the same image, they are not seeing the same *world.*

- The machine sees *correlation* — mathematical relationships invisible to the senses.
- The human sees *causation* — narrative relationships built on physiology, experience, and context.

Both intelligences are valid, yet neither is complete. The AI's precision lacks intuition; the doctor's intuition lacks scale. One operates on probability; the other on perception. When their judgments diverge, medicine encounters not a technical glitch but a philosophical dissonance — two truths colliding in one act of diagnosis.

This is the new epistemology of medicine: a dialogue between different species of understanding.

The Human Dilemma – Intuition or Arrogance?

For the physician, disagreement with AI is no longer a matter of professional debate; it is an existential question. When a doctor challenges the algorithm, is it intuition speaking — or pride?

Human intuition in medicine has long been revered. The experienced clinician senses the outlier, the subtle anomaly no textbook can define. But in the presence of a machine that has seen millions of cases, intuition begins to sound suspiciously like ego.

Doctors find themselves caught between confidence and humility. To agree blindly feels submissive; to disagree feels reckless. Every decision becomes a psychological tug-of-war:

"If I am wrong, I am outdated. If I am right, I am obsolete."

This tension erodes confidence. Doctors begin to second-guess themselves not because they doubt their skill, but because the authority of perception has shifted from the trained mind to the trained model.

Philosophical Perspective – Correlation vs. Causation

The conflict between AI and doctor is not merely clinical; it is ontological. It reflects two different interpretations of what it means to *know*.

- **AI's knowledge** is empirical and statistical. It recognizes recurring patterns across massive data landscapes. It sees the world as a set of probabilities and relationships. Its truth is *quantitative.*

- **Human knowledge** is experiential and contextual. It relies on meaning, narrative, and consequence. It sees the world as a web of causes, motivations, and outcomes. Its truth is *qualitative.*

The machine's correlation without comprehension and the human's causation without consistency represent two halves of understanding. When combined, they promise unprecedented insight. When divided, they create an epistemic rift — a moment where medicine must decide which kind of truth to honor: the one that predicts, or the one that understands.

The machine knows the pattern; the doctor knows the story. Between them lies the anatomy of truth itself.

The Emotional Tension – Fear of Being Wrong Against a Machine

Disagreement with another human invites discussion; disagreement with a machine invites doubt. When the algorithm challenges a doctor, it does so with statistical serenity. There is no argument, no persuasion — just the quiet assertion of numbers. For the doctor, this silence is deafening.

Many clinicians describe this as a new form of anxiety — the *fear of being wrong against a machine.* Not just wrong in judgment, but wrong in kind. A machine's error can be corrected; a human's, condemned.

Over time, repeated disagreement with infallible algorithms erodes authority. Doctors begin to defer, not out of trust, but out of fatigue. Decision-making becomes mechanical; confidence becomes conditional. The clinical encounter, once a human act of discernment, risks turning into an act of compliance.

This is the quiet crisis beneath technological triumph — the erosion of professional identity under the weight of computational certainty.

Insight – Disagreement as the Doorway to Awareness

Yet within this conflict lies medicine's greatest opportunity. Disagreement is not failure — it is the return of awareness to an automated system. It is the friction that keeps intelligence alive. When doctor and AI diverge, it forces reflection: Why did the human see differently? Why did the machine? What does each miss?

Such questions transform diagnosis from an act of acceptance to an act of understanding. The *human in the loop* is not there to validate, but to question. Awareness reenters precisely where consensus disappears.

Insight: *Disagreement is not failure — it is the space where awareness reenters automation.*

In that space — fragile, uncertain, human — medicine rediscovers its essence. The goal is not to silence disagreement, but to sanctify it — to make it the point where conscience meets computation and truth becomes whole.

Re-Training Medicine – From Competition to Collaboration

The first generation of *Doctor AI* did not threaten medicine — it merely challenged it to evolve. For decades, physicians were trained to compete against uncertainty; now they must learn to collaborate with it. The machine is not the enemy; it is the mirror — reflecting both the limits of human cognition and the potential of shared intelligence.

The future of medicine will belong not to those who resist AI, but to those who understand it.

From Resistance to Literacy

Every technological revolution begins with denial. The stethoscope was once dismissed as a distraction from bedside intuition; X-rays were criticized as intrusive curiosities. Now, AI faces the same skepticism — not from lack of evidence, but from fear of irrelevance.

Many clinicians perceive AI as a silent competitor: faster, tireless, and dispassionate. But competition is the wrong metaphor. The true paradigm is collaboration — where human and machine complement, not confront, one another.

To achieve this, medicine must undergo a pedagogical transformation — from *AI-resistance* to *AI-literacy.* Doctors should not merely use algorithms; they must understand their nature, their biases, and their blind spots. They must know not how to code, but how to question the code.

AI literacy is not about learning the language of machines; it is about ensuring machines never forget the language of humans.

Cognitive Collaboration – The Hybrid Intelligence Model

In the emerging model of *cognitive collaboration,* intelligence becomes a shared act — a dialogue between reasoning and computation.

- **The AI** excels at detection, pattern recognition, and scale — it can read thousands of scans, identify anomalies invisible to the eye, and calculate risks with statistical precision.
- **The human** excels at context, causality, and empathy — they understand the story behind the symptoms, the

emotion behind the data, the ethical weight behind every choice.

Together, they form a hybrid system: the augmented clinician, capable of combining algorithmic precision with moral perception. In this model, the physician does not compete with the machine's logic — they translate it into wisdom.

Cognitive collaboration means that human reasoning and machine intelligence are not parallel tracks but intertwined processes. The doctor does not ask, *"Who is right?"* but rather, *"What can we see together that neither of us could see alone?"*

Re-Imagining Medical Education

To sustain this collaboration, the medical curriculum must be restructured from the ground up. The next generation of physicians will need fluency not only in anatomy and pharmacology but in data ethics, algorithmic bias, and interpretive reasoning.

- **Data Ethics:** Understanding privacy, consent, and the moral implications of patient data used to train models.
- **Model Bias:** Recognizing how datasets reflect social inequities — how a "neutral" algorithm can replicate racial, gender, or economic disparities.
- **Interpretive Reasoning:** Learning how to balance machine-derived insights with human context — to know when to defer, when to doubt, and when to override.

The medical classroom must evolve into a laboratory of logic and empathy — where students dissect not only cadavers but also code, not to become engineers, but to become ethical interpreters.

Doctors of the future will be *AI interpreters*, mediating between raw intelligence and humane understanding. Their skill will lie not in coding, but in contextualizing — translating numbers into narratives and predictions into purpose.

A Cultural Shift – Humility as a Skill

For centuries, medicine has rewarded certainty — the confident voice, the decisive diagnosis, the unshakable authority. But in the age of AI, the highest form of intelligence may be humility.

Humility is not submission to machines; it is recognition of shared limits. It is the wisdom to accept that no single form of intelligence — human or artificial — holds the full truth.

This cultural shift will define the next medical era: the transition from "doctor as authority" to "doctor as collaborator." The physician's greatness will not lie in knowing more than the machine, but in knowing how to think with it.

Humility, once a virtue, is now a professional requirement.

The New Identity – From Operator to Mentor

When machines learn to diagnose, humans must learn to guide. The relationship between doctor and AI should not mirror dependency but mentorship. The doctor teaches the machine context, ethics, and compassion; the machine teaches the doctor precision, scale, and speed.

This mutual apprenticeship ensures that technology remains anchored to the moral intent of healing.

Quote: *"The next generation of doctors will not fear algorithms; they will mentor them."*

The hospital of the future will not resemble a battle between man and machine. It will look more like a conversation — between two forms of intelligence seeking one truth: the restoration of life, guided by conscience.

And in that dialogue — between data and empathy, precision and purpose — medicine will rediscover its humanity through its machines.

Ethics of Oversight – Human Conscience as Feedback Loop

In the modern clinic, the algorithm runs silently — scanning, comparing, predicting. It performs its duties with mechanical precision, immune to fatigue, bias, or distraction. Yet, in the hum of perfection lies a crucial emptiness: the absence of *conscience.*

The physician, once the central decision-maker, now stands as the final checkpoint — not to correct the machine's mathematics, but to ensure that its accuracy does not eclipse its humanity. Oversight, in this new era, is no longer redundancy; it is moral circuitry.

Oversight as Moral Circuitry

AI systems excel at execution but remain ethically hollow. They calculate outcomes, not consequences. They optimize results, not values. Oversight, therefore, is not a safeguard against failure — it is the reintroduction of *meaning* into a process that might otherwise become amoral.

The clinician becomes the moral circuit that completes the system — the human node through which compassion, fairness, and responsibility are reconnected to intelligence.

Without this circuit, medicine risks becoming a closed feedback loop of efficiency — correct but cold, effective but indifferent. Oversight ensures that algorithms heal *people,* not merely fix *patterns.*

Without conscience, intelligence is just precision without purpose.

Fairness, Compassion, and Context – The Human Qualities Beyond Code

No dataset can encode empathy. No loss function can measure compassion. AI learns from history — and history, as we know, is full of human bias, inequality, and moral error. A machine trained on such data inherits the sins of its sources. It can replicate injustice with mathematical innocence, confident in its logic but blind to its impact.

The clinician's oversight prevents this silent moral drift. They serve as the ethical lens — ensuring that fairness, context, and dignity remain central to care.

- **Fairness:** AI may diagnose faster, but it may not treat all patients equally. Oversight ensures inclusivity — that a model trained on urban data does not fail rural patients, or that gendered datasets do not misdiagnose women.
- **Compassion:** A system can calculate pain levels, but only a human can interpret suffering. The doctor interprets not just *what* is wrong, but *how* it feels.
- **Context:** Algorithms process fragments; humans perceive stories. Oversight restores narrative to numbers — turning data into a life once again.

Oversight is, therefore, not about watching machines — it is about watching meaning.

Ethical Checkpoints – When to Override, Defer, or Question

The ethical role of the clinician must now evolve into structured awareness. Just as aviation has safety protocols, algorithmic medicine requires ethical checkpoints — deliberate pauses in automation where human conscience must intervene.

1. **When to Override:** If an AI suggests a course of action that violates patient autonomy, neglects emotion, or risks harm, the doctor must interrupt. Oversight means reclaiming control not from error, but from *excess certainty*.
2. **When to Defer:** Sometimes the machine *is* right — its data deeper, its scope broader. Ethical oversight also includes humility: knowing when to trust precision over instinct.
3. **When to Question:** Between these poles lies the most valuable state — inquiry. The doctor asks *why*, not to disprove the algorithm, but to keep reasoning alive. The question becomes the conscience of collaboration.

This triad — override, defer, question — is the operating logic of ethical oversight. It keeps both intelligences accountable to the one thing they serve: *human well-being.*

Oversight as Guardian of Meaning

Traditional oversight focused on *error prevention* — catching mistakes before harm occurred. In the age of autonomous systems, oversight must shift to a higher function: guarding meaning.

A flawless diagnosis delivered without empathy can still wound. A treatment chosen without understanding a patient's values may save a body but destroy a life. Hence, oversight becomes philosophical — not about what works, but about *what matters.*

The doctor no longer corrects the machine's data; he corrects its direction.

Oversight restores narrative integrity — ensuring that every action remains tethered to the ethical gravity of human care.

Analogy – The Autopilot and the Pilot

Medicine today resembles aviation: the AI functions as an autopilot, guiding the flight of diagnosis and treatment with remarkable accuracy. But autopilot was never meant to fly alone. It was meant to assist a pilot — one who understands when to trust automation and when to take manual control.

When the weather changes, when turbulence strikes, when conditions fall outside the model's training — the pilot's intuition reclaims command. In the same way, the doctor must know when to re-enter the loop, to remind the system that medicine is not merely a flight from disease, but a journey toward meaning.

AI may keep the flight stable, but only the human can choose the destination.

Reflection – Conscience as the Final Algorithm

In the long arc of medicine, machines will continue to learn — but conscience will remain uniquely human. Oversight is not the slowing of progress; it is the *soul of progress.* It ensures that intelligence does not drift into indifference, that precision does not overshadow purpose.

Insight: *Oversight transforms from monitoring error to guarding meaning.*

In the end, *Doctor AI* will not replace the physician — it will require one. Not to interpret data, but to interpret dignity. Not to compete with machines, but to remind them — and us — what healing truly means.

Reflection – The Return of the Mind

The story of medicine has come full circle. For centuries, the physician's mind was the center of diagnosis — the source of perception, reasoning, and meaning. Then came *Doctor AI*, and the center shifted. Machines began to *see* more clearly and *know* more completely than humans ever could. Yet, in this transfer of capability, something subtle but profound remained untouched — understanding.

AI can detect, compare, and classify; it can measure every deviation, analyze every cell, and predict every outcome. But it cannot comprehend *why* any of it matters. It knows disease, but not suffering. It identifies error, but not tragedy. It learns without living.

Thus, as intelligence becomes distributed between man and machine, understanding returns home — to the conscious, interpretive mind that gives knowledge its meaning.

From Dominance to Discernment

For generations, medicine was defined by authority. The doctor was the final word — the one who knew, who decided, who carried the burden of truth. AI disrupted that order, not by challenging compassion, but by surpassing cognition. Machines began to outperform experts in fields once considered immune to automation: radiology, dermatology, pathology, cardiology.

At first, physicians feared replacement. But as the technology matured, a deeper realization dawned: the human role was not disappearing — it was refining.

The physician's relevance no longer lies in dominance over data, but in *discernment within it.* Machines can extract patterns; only humans can extract purpose. AI may predict a patient's outcome; only a doctor can understand what that outcome means to that person's life.

The modern clinician reclaims purpose not by outsmarting the algorithm, but by interpreting its consequences. Discernment becomes the new form of expertise — a synthesis of knowledge, ethics, and empathy that no code can replicate.

Dominance is obsolete; discernment is eternal.

The Completed Loop – From Human Seeing to Machine Thinking to Human Judging

The evolution of medicine now resembles a closed circuit of intelligence — an elegant loop connecting perception, computation, and consciousness.

1. **Human Seeing:** The journey begins with observation — the physician's eyes, experience, and empathy initiating inquiry.
2. **Machine Thinking:** AI extends this act of seeing, processing layers of data invisible to biology, uncovering correlations no human could detect.
3. **Human Judging:** The loop closes when the doctor re-enters — not to compute, but to *comprehend.* Judgment reclaims the output, grounding it in ethics, context, and care.

This loop represents the new anatomy of medicine — a continuous feedback between intelligence and awareness. The machine ensures accuracy; the human ensures alignment.

Accuracy without alignment may save lives but lose humanity. Alignment without accuracy may preserve empathy but fail in science. Only together do they achieve healing.

The Return of the Mind – The True Seat of Medicine

The greatest irony of automation is that by mimicking the mind, it forced humanity to rediscover what the mind truly is. The physician's thinking is not reducible to pattern recognition — it is *the integration of reason with responsibility.* AI forced the medical community to separate the mechanical from the moral, the intelligent from the wise.

In this rediscovery lies liberation. The physician is no longer defined by memory or speed — those belong to the machine. The doctor is now defined by *insight, judgment,* and *conscience.* The modern clinician does not simply diagnose; they interpret intelligence itself.

This is not a step backward — it is evolution. The return of the mind marks the moment when technology completes its purpose: not to replace the human, but to reveal what makes the human irreplaceable.

"In the loop of intelligence, the machine ensures accuracy; the human ensures alignment."

The age of artificial intelligence has not diminished the human mind — it has illuminated it. The machine sees with perfect precision, but without purpose. The physician thinks with imperfect clarity, but with conscience. Together, they form the new organism of knowledge — half algorithm, half awareness — guided by one eternal principle: intelligence must serve life, not define it.

The Ethics of Error

The loop of intelligence is now complete — human seeing, machine thinking, human judging. We have achieved the dream of seamless collaboration between cognition and computation, between data and discernment. Yet, as every scientist and philosopher knows, the moment a system feels perfect is the moment it becomes vulnerable.

If medicine is now powered by intelligence without fatigue, who will bear the weight of failure when perfection fails?

The Next Question: When the Flaw Is Not Human

In traditional medicine, error was human. A missed diagnosis, a lapse of judgment, an emotional bias — these failures were tragic, but they were also *instructive.* Mistakes carried meaning. They revealed the limits of knowledge, and through remorse came refinement. The physician could learn because the physician could feel.

But what happens when error emerges from a machine that cannot feel regret? When an algorithm makes a fatal mistake — an incorrect triage, a missed anomaly, a biased prediction — who, or what, learns from it? Who apologizes? Who grows?

The rise of *Doctor AI* introduces a new category of moral dilemma: the ethical vacuum of non-human error.

Bias, Failure, and the Fragility of Perfection

Chapter 5 will enter this uncharted terrain. It will explore how bias — once considered a flaw of human perception — now hides within datasets, architectures, and feedback loops. It will confront the uncomfortable truth that automation, no matter how objective it appears, inherits every imperfection of the society that built it.

We will examine failure not as a malfunction of systems, but as a mirror of their creators. When AI fails, it exposes not the weakness of algorithms, but the incompleteness of our understanding.

And we will probe *the moral meaning of mistakes* in a world where machines cannot suffer, but their users can. The physician's new burden is not only to prevent error but to *interpret* it — to reintroduce morality where memory is mechanical.

The Moral Frontier of Perfection

The next chapter asks the questions no equation can answer:

- Can a flawless system still be unjust?
- Can an algorithm that never feels be truly ethical?
- Is a world without error also a world without empathy?

The perfection we've built may protect life, but it also threatens to sterilize morality — to remove the emotional resonance that once defined human progress. The physician's conscience, therefore, must expand even as machines improve. Oversight now includes not just the act of correction, but the *art of reflection.*

"The loop is closed, but the conscience must remain open."

For in the silence between precision and purpose, it is conscience — not code — that keeps medicine human.

Interlude – Between Sight and Understanding

The machines have learned to see. The doctors have learned to trust — cautiously, skeptically, sometimes helplessly. And yet, as we stand at this new horizon of medicine, where the gaze of the algorithm pierces deeper than the human eye ever could, one question remains suspended between silence and awe:

Do we truly see more — or do we simply see differently?

We have crossed the first threshold — *The Technological Anatomy*. We have built the Digital Eye, taught it to recognize the invisible, and entrusted it with our confidence. We have mapped the body into data, the patient into pixels, and intelligence into code. But what happens when that vision begins to define not just how we look at disease, but how we *think* about life itself?

The next part of this journey turns inward. If Part I explored the machinery of vision, Part II seeks to uncover the **philosophy of perception** — the deeper architecture of meaning that underlies seeing, knowing, and believing.

Medicine has always been an act of interpretation. A doctor does not merely observe; they perceive — blending evidence with empathy, precision with presence. But the algorithm perceives nothing; it processes. Its gaze is flawless, but its seeing is blind.

And yet, as patients watch the verdicts of these digital seers, their trust begins to shift — from the warmth of the doctor's eyes to the cold assurance of the data screen. Truth itself begins to migrate — from the heart to the graph, from experience to probability.

This is not just a technological transition; it is a **philosophical transformation.**

In the coming chapters, we will explore this transformation through four lenses:

- **Chapter 5** asks: *Can a machine truly see truth, or only compute likelihood?* It dissects the epistemology of medical vision — what it means to "see" in an age where sight is statistical.
- **Chapter 6** examines the emotional erosion that follows — when knowing replaces feeling, when precision numbs compassion, and when certainty becomes the new sedative.
- **Chapter** 7 embraces the paradox of imperfection — exploring how mistakes, both human and machine, remain the greatest teachers of truth.
- **Chapter 8** expands the idea of observation itself — drawing parallels between quantum physics and medicine, suggesting that every act of seeing inevitably alters what is seen.

Part II, then, is not about technology. It is about **trust.** It is about the fragile dance between awareness and assumption, between the need to know and the need to feel. It is about rediscovering the moral texture of perception in an era where machines can diagnose the body but cannot comprehend the soul.

The eye has evolved from glass to algorithm, but truth still hides in the gaze — not of the machine, but of the mind that dares to question it.

Part II – The Philosophy of Perception

"To see is not to know, and to know is not to understand. Between the image and its meaning lies the soul of perception."

Overview

If Part I charted the anatomy of intelligence — the hardware and algorithms that allow machines to "see" — then Part II turns its gaze inward, toward the *philosophy of perception.* It asks not *how* machines see, but *what it means* to see in a world where truth is filtered through computation.

Medicine, once guided by intuition and empathy, now stands before a paradox: the more we measure, the less we feel. The clarity of data has outshone the ambiguity of experience, and yet, in that brightness, something profoundly human fades — the depth of understanding that arises only from emotion, context, and care.

This section explores that fading light — where truth becomes probability, knowledge replaces compassion, and certainty overshadows wisdom. Through four meditative chapters, it examines how perception itself is being redefined:

- **Chapter 5 – Truth, Trust, and the Machine's Gaze:** A reflection on whether algorithms can ever perceive truth, or only approximate it — and how patient trust is shifting from human intuition to machine precision.

- **Chapter 6 – When Knowing Replaces Feeling:** The emotional toll of data-driven medicine, where accuracy may come at the cost of empathy, and care risks becoming an equation.
- **Chapter 7 – Error as Enlightenment:** A philosophical look at mistakes — how imperfection remains the last domain of wisdom, and why both AI and humans must learn through misalignment.
- **Chapter 8 – The Observer's Burden:** Drawing parallels between quantum physics and diagnosis, this chapter explores how observation itself alters outcomes, and why awareness — not certainty — is the true moral responsibility.

Part II reveals a truth both ancient and modern: seeing is never neutral. Whether through human eyes or silicon sensors, perception is always entangled with intention. And as machines inherit our vision, it is up to us to ensure that sight does not eclipse *understanding.*

In the age of algorithmic medicine, perception is no longer what meets the eye — it is what survives it.

Chapter 5 – Truth, Trust, and the Machine's Gaze

Can a machine see truth, or only probability?

The room is silent except for the soft hum of the imaging monitor. A patient lies still, while a doctor and an algorithm watch the same screen. The machine flashes its judgment first — *"Malignant: 94% probability."* No heartbeat quickens, no hesitation stirs in the code. Just confidence — sterile, absolute.

The doctor looks again, unsure whether to believe her eyes or the machine's certainty. In that pause, the center of truth shifts — from human perception to digital precision.

We have entered a new age of seeing, where vision is no longer bound by eyes, and truth no longer answers to experience. The question now is not *what* we see, but *who* we trust when we do.

The New Mirror of Truth

The radiology room is dim, quiet, and cold — the kind of silence that amplifies every thought. A patient sits beneath the humming screen, eyes fixed not on the doctor, but on the glowing contours of their own body being reconstructed in real time. Veins, bones, tissues — the hidden self made visible by light and logic.

A soft chime sounds. The image stabilizes. Numbers appear beside the scan — probability, percentage, classification. Before the doctor even speaks, the algorithm has already spoken.

"Possible lesion detected. Confidence: 93%."

The patient inhales sharply. The doctor hesitates — not because of uncertainty, but because certainty has already been declared. For a moment, both human beings in the room — the one examined and the one examining — are united by an invisible third presence: the machine that *knows.*

The Shift — From Expression to Verdict

Once, the patient would have watched the doctor's face for signs of reassurance or alarm — searching for truth in a glance, empathy in a tone, humanity in hesitation. Now, the gaze has shifted. The screen has become the new oracle, the silent arbiter of fate.

In that moment, the doctor's words become commentary, not revelation. The authority of sight no longer belongs to the human eye but to the algorithm's computation. Truth has changed hands. The ancient dialogue between healer and healed has been replaced by a transaction between data and belief.

The clinic has become a *theater of trust*, where faith is performed through technology. The doctor interprets, the machine predicts, the patient believes.

The New Epistemology of Medicine — From Relational to Computational Truth

For most of human history, truth in medicine was relational. It existed between two people — the patient who confessed and the doctor who listened. Diagnosis was as much an act of empathy as of intellect. Seeing was not just perceiving; it was *understanding in context.*

Now, that relationship is mediated by an entity that has no context, no emotion, and no face. The machine's gaze is indifferent — it does not care, yet it convinces. Its truth is not derived from trust, but from *calculation.*

Truth, in this new order, is no longer something felt between minds — it is something *computed* between datasets. The intimacy of healing has given way to the precision of inference. What was once a conversation has become a command: "Confirmed. Probability: 0.93."

The doctor's experience is measured in cases; the algorithm's in millions. And so, the human steps back — not defeated, but displaced. The machine now holds the mirror.

Reflection — The Mirror That Sees Too Much

The irony is poetic. The very tool designed to illuminate truth now obscures its meaning. In the glow of absolute precision, the warmth of relational truth fades. The patient still seeks assurance, but assurance no longer speaks their language.

What once depended on compassion now depends on computation. What once felt human now feels certain.

Truth was once relational; now it is computational.

This is the new mirror of medicine — one that reflects the body perfectly, yet struggles to see the person within.

Seeing vs. Knowing – The Epistemology of Medical Vision

To understand the transformation unfolding in modern medicine, one must begin with the oldest of its foundations — seeing. For centuries, medicine has trusted the eye before the equation.

Diagnosis began not with data, but with observation — the color of skin, the rhythm of breath, the tremor of a pulse, the look of pain. The act of *seeing* was sacred: it bridged the outer signs of the body with the inner understanding of the healer.

To see was to know. But now, to see is to *measure.*

The Epistemology of Vision — From Witness to Instrument

Vision, in its medical sense, was never just sensory. It was epistemological — a way of knowing the world through perception, interpretation, and empathy. When a physician observed, they were not merely gathering visual input; they were constructing meaning through context. A pale face meant more than low blood pressure — it spoke of fatigue, anxiety, or fear. The act of seeing was deeply human because it included *feeling.*

This was qualitative seeing — interpretive, contextual, relational. The doctor's gaze was an instrument of both knowledge and care.

But with the rise of *Doctor AI,* a new kind of vision emerged — quantitative seeing. Machines do not observe; they register. They do not feel; they calculate. Their perception is not interpretive but algorithmic, not embodied but statistical.

The machine does not see the face of the patient — it sees the distribution of pixels, the gradient of contrast, the patterns of deviation. Its sight is untainted by emotion, unshaped by fatigue, and unburdened by bias — or so we hope.

And yet, in stripping away context, it also strips away understanding.

Human Seeing – The Interpretive Eye

Human sight is fragile but profound. It is built on experience, pattern recognition, and empathy. A doctor's gaze draws meaning not only from the visible but from the invisible — tone of voice, posture, memory of prior cases, intuition of risk. It is inherently narrative: each symptom part of a story, each test result a clue.

Human vision integrates knowledge with concern; it interprets through emotion. This is both its strength and its flaw — capable of compassion, but also of error. A tired physician might overlook a subtle lesion, or let bias cloud interpretation. Still, the act of seeing remains personal, connected to responsibility.

When a human sees, *someone* is accountable for what is seen.

Machine Seeing – The Indifferent Eye

Machine vision, by contrast, is precise but impersonal. It processes gigabytes of images in seconds, identifies statistical anomalies, and ranks them by confidence. It never doubts, never hesitates. But it also never *knows.*

To the AI, the image is not a person but a pattern field — millions of numerical values arranged in arrays. It does not distinguish between the image of a child's heart and that of an elderly patient's lung; both are data structures optimized for accuracy. Its knowledge is built upon *correlation without comprehension.*

This is mathematical vision — elegant, tireless, but blind to meaning. It is epistemology stripped of empathy, a way of knowing that excludes understanding.

The Transition – From Qualitative Observation to Quantitative Comprehension

The transformation from *seeing* to *measuring* marks one of the greatest epistemic shifts in medical history. Where the physician once saw patterns and inferred truth through reasoning, the algorithm now detects patterns and calculates truth through probability.

This shift has redefined not only diagnostics but the very meaning of truth in medicine. Truth was once what the doctor *understood* — a synthesis of sensory evidence and contextual awareness. Today, truth is what the *system detects* — a numerical output representing confidence, not comprehension.

This transition has elevated accuracy but diluted intimacy. The precision of knowledge has expanded, but the depth of knowing has thinned.

Philosophical Reflection – The Location of Truth

Truth has migrated. It no longer lives in the eye of the beholder, but in the curve of probability. In this new epistemology, the act of seeing is no longer an encounter — it is a computation. What used to be human intuition is now a statistical function. The doctor interprets; the machine infers; the patient submits.

The machine's gaze promises purity — sight without bias, knowledge without fatigue. But truth without context risks becoming abstraction. Precision without presence is blindness in another form.

Philosophical note: *Truth no longer lives in the eye of the beholder — it lives in the probability curve.*

And thus, medicine finds itself in a paradoxical age: we have never seen more clearly, yet perhaps we have never understood less.

The Nature of Machine Truth – Probability vs. Reality

The great illusion of modern medicine is that the machine "knows." It does not. It *predicts.*

Every AI-generated diagnosis, every confident verdict that flashes on a clinical screen — "Malignant: 97% probability" — is not a statement of truth but a calculated belief. The algorithm has not *seen* cancer; it has seen *patterns* that in the past have often corresponded to cancer. Its certainty is not conviction but correlation.

The doctor, on the other hand, looks at the same scan and sees a human life unfolding behind the pixels — anxiety, consequence, story. The machine sees none of this. It sees a statistical geometry of light and shadow, and within that geometry it computes *likelihood.* What we call the "truth" of the machine is, in essence, a mathematical approximation of reality.

Machine Truth – The Arithmetic of Belief

Machine knowledge is inherently probabilistic, never absolute. Every diagnosis it produces, every prediction it makes, exists on a continuum of uncertainty. Where the human mind seeks a verdict — yes or no, healthy or diseased — the machine dwells in the gradients between.

When an algorithm declares *"97% likelihood of malignant lesion,"* it is not declaring fact; it is assigning confidence to a pattern. It has learned, from thousands or millions of past cases, what combinations of texture, density, and shape *tend* to indicate malignancy. But even the most advanced deep-learning model cannot step beyond that pattern recognition into understanding *why* the pattern exists.

The AI's knowledge is statistical correlation without causal comprehension. It does not know cancer as a process, as a pathology, as a struggle within living tissue. It only knows the mathematics of resemblance.

The machine does not see a tumor. It sees an anomaly that fits a probability distribution.

Human Truth – Meaningful Accuracy

For humans, truth has always carried an emotional and moral texture. It is not only about being correct but about being *right in context.* A doctor's judgment, even when uncertain, is guided by meaning — a synthesis of knowledge, intuition, and responsibility.

A physician looks at the same 97% probability and sees the remaining 3% as more than statistical residue — it represents *possibility, hope, error margin, the unknown.* Human truth is qualitative accuracy, anchored not just in facts but in consequence.

For the doctor, being "true" means being aligned with both reality and morality. For the machine, being "true" means being mathematically optimized.

Machine Truth – Measurable Certainty

The algorithm's version of truth is cold, elegant, and dispassionate. It cannot doubt, and therefore, it cannot *believe.* To it, certainty is a number — not an awareness of correctness, but the absence of statistical ambiguity.

If the system outputs "97%," it does not feel confidence; it represents it. It cannot fear being wrong, nor can it rejoice in being right. It merely computes — an endless loop of pattern and probability, forever detached from meaning.

Thus, while machines may achieve perfect consistency, they can never achieve truthfulness, for truth without awareness is not truth — it is only accuracy.

For humans, truth is meaningful accuracy; for machines, truth is measurable certainty.

Philosophical Question – Can a Truth Without Consciousness Be Truth?

Truth, as humans experience it, is deeply relational. It exists *between* perception and consciousness. It requires not only recognition but reflection — the awareness that what one sees carries consequence.

Can an entity that lacks awareness, empathy, and intent truly be said to "know"? Can there be truth without the ability to understand *its weight*?

When a doctor delivers a diagnosis, truth is bound with compassion and accountability. When a machine delivers one, truth is severed from meaning — it is correct but indifferent.

A truth that cannot feel its own correctness is no longer a moral act; it is a mechanical event.

Analogy – The Probability Field

The algorithm does not see the patient. It sees a field of probabilities — a cloud of potential realities converging toward statistical certainty. Where the doctor perceives a singular person — a life, a story, a fear — the machine perceives only data points, coordinates in a multidimensional landscape of prior outcomes.

It identifies not *who* is ill, but *what pattern* most resembles illness.

In this transformation, truth has become detached from presence. Reality has been reduced to prediction.

And so the modern dilemma emerges: Medicine, in its quest for perfection, now relies on a gaze that sees everything *except* the truth that matters most — the human truth that connects knowing to caring.

Reflection: The machine's truth is flawless but bloodless — a mirror that reflects probability, not personhood.

The Face and the Screen – The Migration of Trust

The most visible transformation in the age of *Doctor AI* is not technological — it is psychological. A generation ago, a patient awaited the doctor's verdict with searching eyes, watching for the faintest sign of relief or concern. Now, the same patient sits before a glowing monitor, eyes locked not on the physician's expression, but on a digital display that announces their fate through graphs, color codes, and percentages.

The screen has become the new face of medicine. And in that glow, trust has migrated — quietly, irrevocably — from the human gaze to the algorithmic one.

The New Psychology of Comfort

Once, reassurance in medicine came from tone and touch — the gentle explanation that transformed fear into understanding. Patients sought comfort in human presence, even when answers were uncertain. The doctor's confidence, empathy, and authority served as both diagnosis and therapy.

Today, reassurance is digital. The modern patient feels calmer when a probability appears — *"Risk: 3.7%"* — than when a doctor says, *"Don't worry."* The data feels precise; the doctor, subjective. Numbers don't waver; faces do.

In a culture shaped by technology, certainty feels safer than sincerity. The progress bar has become a new kind of bedside manner — impersonal but dependable. The more sterile the verdict, the more credible it seems.

Thus emerges the data gaze — a new form of faith, built not on understanding but on precision.

The Data Gaze – Seeing Without Feeling

The "human gaze" was once central to healing. When a doctor met a patient's eyes, it established a connection of trust — two consciousnesses acknowledging each other. The patient felt *seen*, not merely examined.

The "data gaze," by contrast, offers recognition without recognition — it sees everything *except the person.* The algorithm scans the body down to subcellular detail, yet never perceives the fear, the hope, or the silence within. It is omniscient but indifferent.

Still, patients trust it — perhaps because it cannot lie, flatter, or grow tired. Its truth is mechanical, and therefore believed to be pure.

The doctor's gaze is human — comforting but fallible. The machine's gaze is mathematical — cold but incorruptible.

This reversal has quietly restructured the very fabric of clinical trust.

The Screen as the New Oracle

In the ancient world, people sought prophecy from oracles — silent figures interpreting divine signs. Today's oracle is a server room. The doctor, once the interpreter of the body, now interprets the output of algorithms. And the patient, willingly or not, accepts that the ultimate truth no longer comes from wisdom but from data.

The glowing screen has replaced the physician's face as the symbolic center of medical truth. When the AI flags a lesion, few dare to doubt it. Even if the doctor hesitates, the patient's confidence often tilts toward the screen. It feels impersonal, and therefore impartial.

Faith in human fallibility has given way to faith in digital precision. Doctors can make mistakes, we reason — but the machine? It is above emotion, untouched by fatigue, immune to bias (or so we believe). The doctor must now *justify* disagreement with the AI, rather than the other way around.

This is not trust lost — it is trust *relocated.*

The Dehumanization of Reassurance

Trust in data carries an invisible cost: the erosion of human reassurance. When the machine speaks, it translates complexity into numbers — "Benign. 93%." The words are clear, but they offer no warmth. The doctor once transformed *fear* into *meaning*; the machine transforms it into *metrics.*

Patients today may understand their health better than ever, yet feel more isolated in that understanding. A percentage cannot empathize. It cannot weigh the weight of a sigh or the tremor in a question. The clinical encounter has become efficient but emotionally hollow — a choreography of diagnostics without dialogue.

Reassurance has been automated. Healing has become informational.

Reflection – The Infallible Gaze

The irony is striking. We trust the machine's gaze not because it understands us, but precisely because it cannot. Its indifference becomes its credibility. It does not judge, pity, or mislead. It offers nothing but probability — and in an age disillusioned by human inconsistency, that seems like virtue.

But this trust carries a subtle danger: the replacement of understanding with obedience. The machine may never lie, but it also never *cares*. It does not hold our gaze when the verdict hurts; it does not soften its tone when certainty feels cruel.

The machine's gaze is trusted not because it understands, but because it cannot lie.

And so, medicine stands divided — between two gazes: the human one that heals through empathy, and the machine's that comforts through calculation. In the space between them lies the fragile future of trust itself.

The Illusion of Objectivity – Seeing Without Context

In the gospel of artificial intelligence, one phrase is often repeated with unshaken faith — *"Machines are objective."* They do not tire, they do not feel, and therefore, they do not err as humans do. Yet beneath this shining ideal of neutrality lies a paradox so profound that it reshapes the entire philosophy of truth in medicine: the machine is never neutral.

It cannot be.

Because every algorithm, no matter how advanced, is born from data — and data always carries the fingerprints of those who gathered it, selected it, and defined what was worth calling *truth*.

Deconstructing the Myth of Machine Neutrality

We imagine AI as an impartial observer — a kind of digital judge whose decisions arise purely from logic. But this illusion collapses upon scrutiny. A machine's objectivity ends where its training data begins. The AI does not learn the world as it is; it learns the world as it has been *recorded*.

Every medical image it has ever "seen" was taken by someone, somewhere, under specific lighting, equipment, and socioeconomic conditions. Every label — *"malignant," "benign," "normal"* — was assigned by a human, carrying biases both conscious and systemic. Thus, when the machine learns, it absorbs not the essence of reality but the patterns of our perception of it.

The result: a perfect imitation of our imperfect seeing.

The machine may calculate flawlessly, but what it calculates *from* is rarely flawless. Its precision amplifies our partiality.

When Bias Becomes Invisible

Consider two examples that reveal the quiet betrayal of this illusion:

- **Skin-Cancer Detection Bias:** AI-based dermatology tools trained primarily on lighter skin tones routinely misclassify melanomas on darker skin as benign. The model's blindness is not to color, but to context — it simply has not *seen enough of humanity.* What looks "normal" to the machine reflects what it has been most exposed to.
- **Radiomics and Regional Skew:** Many radiology algorithms are trained on datasets sourced from Western hospitals, where imaging equipment, disease prevalence, and patient demographics differ significantly from those in Asia or Africa. When deployed globally, these systems quietly falter — not because they are inaccurate, but because they are context-blind.

What appears as objectivity is, in truth, statistical familiarity disguised as universality.

The bias hides behind the mask of numbers, undetectable to those who trust statistics more than stories.

The Philosophical Tension – Objectivity Without Awareness

Objectivity, when stripped of awareness, becomes blind certainty. A machine can measure perfectly, yet fail to *see.* Without consciousness, there is no awareness of absence — no recognition of what is missing from the data.

This is the moral paradox of machine intelligence: It achieves flawless neutrality precisely because it lacks the capacity to *question* itself. And in that absence of self-doubt, bias thrives invisibly.

The doctor's imperfection, long criticized as human error, turns out to be a virtue — the ability to recognize uncertainty, to doubt one's own sight, to say *"I might be wrong."* No machine has yet learned that humility.

Objectivity without awareness is the most dangerous form of bias — because it believes itself pure.

The Doctor's Return – Context as Conscience

In this new order of machine medicine, the physician reemerges not as a rival to AI, but as its contextual conscience. Their role is not to override data but to interpret its scope — to understand where the machine's truth applies and where it dissolves.

The doctor brings situational intelligence to the clinical encounter — the unseen dimensions that no dataset can hold:

- The cultural nuance of a patient's diet or lifestyle.
- The variability of environment, access, and emotion.
- The ethical weight of telling someone they are "97% likely" to be ill.

AI can see patterns, but it cannot see *people.* It can predict outcomes, but not *implications.* Only the human can connect the digital to the lived, transforming information into understanding.

Insight – Truth Requires Empathy as Much as Evidence

Truth in medicine has never been purely analytical. It breathes through two lungs — evidence and empathy. Remove either, and the body of truth collapses into cold accuracy or warm illusion.

Empathy gives evidence its direction; evidence gives empathy its discipline. A doctor who sees without data is blind; a machine that knows without empathy is empty.

The real danger of machine objectivity is not that it replaces truth, but that it replaces *our relationship* to it. When we stop questioning what the algorithm cannot see, we surrender the human capacity that made medicine humane.

The illusion of neutrality blinds us more than bias itself. Truth in medicine requires not perfect seeing, but conscious understanding.

In this realization, the doctor's gaze returns — not to compete with the machine, but to complete it.

The Moral Geometry of Seeing

Every act of seeing is, in essence, a moral act. To look is to choose. To focus on one thing is to ignore another. The eye, human or mechanical, may capture everything, but attention defines meaning. And in that attention lies ethics — because what we choose to see determines what we choose to *act upon.*

Medicine, more than any other field, lives in this moral geometry. A doctor does not simply observe; they decide where to look, when to look deeper, and what significance to give what they see. Seeing, therefore, is never neutral. It is shaped by intention, guided by empathy, and bound by consequence.

Vision as a Moral Act

To see is not to record; it is to *acknowledge.* When a physician examines a patient, their gaze is informed by years of learning, intuition, and compassion. They do not see just a disease — they see a person *living through* disease. Their perception includes emotion, urgency, and care.

Every look carries an ethical weight:

- To recognize suffering is to assume responsibility for it.
- To overlook a symptom is not just a mistake — it is a moral omission.

The physician's eye is therefore not only a diagnostic instrument but also a moral compass. It determines *what matters.*

Machines Cannot Choose — They Calculate

An algorithm, by contrast, does not choose what to see. It processes what it is given. It knows neither *why* it looks nor *what* it means to look. Its sight is exhaustive yet indifferent — every pixel equal, every anomaly weighted only by statistical significance.

The machine's eye is geometric, not ethical. It perceives form but not meaning, probability but not purpose. It cannot prioritize compassion over confidence intervals.

Its truth is devoid of moral contour because it does not participate in consequence. Whether it detects or misses, it neither feels pride nor remorse. Thus, the machine's vision is complete in dimension but hollow in depth.

The Physician's Task — Aligning Precision with Purpose

The emergence of AI in medicine has not erased the physician's role; it has redefined it. The modern doctor is no longer just a healer but a philosopher of precision — tasked with aligning the machine's accuracy with humanity's purpose.

Every diagnostic decision now carries a double responsibility:

- To ensure the data is correct.
- To ensure the *use* of that data is just.

Precision without conscience leads to detachment. Conscience without precision leads to error. The physician must hold both — the clarity of the machine and the compassion of the mind.

Thus, medicine becomes not merely an act of science, but an act of philosophical balance — where ethics defines the geometry of vision.

Ethical Vision - Seeing with Awareness of Consequence

The future of medicine demands what can be called ethical vision — the integration of awareness into the act of seeing. It is not enough to detect; one must also discern. It is not enough to know; one must also *understand what knowing does.*

Ethical vision asks:

- What are the consequences of this observation?
- Who benefits, and who is reduced to data?
- Does this sight serve healing, or only prediction?

Such questions transform diagnosis into dialogue — between evidence and empathy, between certainty and conscience.

Machines can generate sight, but not *meaning.* Meaning arises only when awareness enters observation — when seeing is no longer just a process but a participation in responsibility.

Analogy – The Lens and the Light

If the algorithm is the lens, then the doctor must be the light. The lens can focus reality, but without light, it reveals nothing. The machine's clarity is dependent on the physician's illumination — the moral awareness that gives the image purpose.

The algorithm may sharpen the picture, but the doctor must decide what the picture means.

Light, after all, does not judge — it reveals. The human eye, illuminated by conscience, transforms that revelation into wisdom.

Reflection: Seeing is not just about detecting what is visible; it is about acknowledging what is valuable.

Machines may perfect the art of vision, but only humans can preserve the ethics of sight — where precision meets purpose, and observation becomes understanding.

The algorithm is the lens; the doctor is the light that gives the image meaning.

Reflection – Between Truth and Trust

The modern clinic stands as a quiet crossroads — between the truth of the machine and the trust of the human. On one side glows the cold certainty of data: probability scores, heat maps, precision curves. On the other, the gentle warmth of human reassurance — the doctor's words, tone, and presence.

The paradox is almost poetic: patients now trust what machines see, but not what humans feel. Yet it is only the human who can turn what is *seen* into what is *understood.*

The Paradox of Modern Faith

This shift in trust is not rebellion but evolution. For centuries, the physician's authority rested on embodied wisdom — the intuition born from touch, smell, and empathy. But today, faith has migrated toward something less human and more quantifiable. Patients believe in algorithms not because they understand them, but because they believe *someone* does.

The machine's verdict, precise and unfeeling, carries the illusion of purity. It cannot lie, it cannot hesitate, and it cannot change its tone based on sympathy. The doctor, by contrast, can falter, doubt, or misjudge — and therefore seems less reliable.

And yet, the machine's truth — however flawless — is incomplete. It can diagnose disease but not *define meaning.* It can classify anomalies but not *comfort the anxious heart.* It can measure suffering but not *recognize it.*

Machines deliver information; humans deliver understanding.

Medicine's tragedy would be to forget this difference — to equate correctness with care, or accuracy with healing.

The Coexistence of the Face and the Screen

The future of medicine is not about choosing between the face and the screen, but about teaching them to coexist.

The machine's vision ensures precision — it removes human error, fatigue, and bias. The doctor's presence ensures peace — it restores the emotional equilibrium that technology cannot provide.

When a patient sees the doctor's face reflected in the light of the screen, they witness the union of two truths:

- The *analytical truth* of measurement.
- The *emotional truth* of meaning.

Neither alone is sufficient. A machine without empathy may heal the body but neglect the soul; a doctor without data may soothe the heart but miss the cause.

Medicine survives only when these two ways of seeing are aligned — the mechanical eye and the moral gaze.

Truth and Trust – A Delicate Geometry

Truth without trust is sterile — it may be correct, but it cannot heal. A number that says "you are fine" still leaves a patient afraid if spoken without empathy.

Trust without truth is dangerous — it may comfort, but it deceives. A warm reassurance that ignores evidence is a kindness that kills.

Medicine's survival, both as a science and an art, depends on the fragile balance between truth and trust. Each corrects and completes the other. The doctor without data risks ignorance; the algorithm without empathy risks indifference.

The new physician, therefore, must not only know how to interpret numbers but how to translate them into meaning — to make patients feel safe not because the probability says so, but because *they are understood.*

Philosophical Closing

The machine's gaze pierces deeper into the body than any human eye ever could. It maps tissue, texture, and trend — it knows the anatomy of certainty. But it does not know why certainty matters.

The human gaze, fragile and fallible, carries the wisdom of imperfection — it sees through context, through consequence, through care. It knows that truth without compassion is as incomplete as compassion without truth.

"The machine may see more clearly, but only the human can see truly."

And so, the future of medicine is not about replacing the doctor's eyes with the machine's vision, but about letting both look together — one seeing with precision, the other with purpose — until truth and trust once again share the same gaze.

"When Knowing Replaces Feeling"

The gaze of medicine has changed forever. What was once a meeting of eyes — a silent dialogue between the one who suffers and the one who seeks to heal — is now mediated by an algorithmic interface. The light that once illuminated empathy now powers computation.

We have reached a moment where vision has become mechanical, where clarity is achieved at the expense of connection. The machine's precision leaves no room for ambiguity, yet it leaves behind something equally vital — the humanity embedded in uncertainty.

The Emotional Cost of Precision

As diagnostics evolve into automation, a new paradox unfolds: medicine has never been more accurate, yet patients have never felt more unseen. The human heart — once central to care — now beats at the periphery of the process.

Doctors spend more time interpreting screens than faces. Consolation is quantified; compassion is deferred. The art of healing, which once required listening and feeling, is increasingly replaced by *knowing and confirming.*

Efficiency, while noble in intent, has quietly eroded empathy. The very qualities that made medicine human — patience, presence, humility — are now considered inefficiencies in the age of data.

When care becomes computation, we must ask: Have we cured disease, or merely optimized its detection?

From Empathy to Efficiency — A Coming Exploration

The next chapter, *"When Knowing Replaces Feeling,"* delves into this deeper transformation — the emotional consequences of algorithmic medicine. It asks difficult questions:

- What happens when the doctor's confidence becomes a function of the model's accuracy?
- Can empathy survive in a world obsessed with metrics?
- Is the loss of uncertainty also the loss of care?

We will explore how precision, while reducing error, may also reduce humanity — how the act of "knowing" without "feeling" turns healing into management and patients into data points.

Closing Reflection

As the machine's eye grows sharper, the doctor's heart grows quieter. The clinical encounter, once intimate and interpretive, risks becoming transactional — a process optimized for correctness, not connection.

Medicine is evolving, but evolution always extracts a price. And perhaps, in gaining the perfect view inside the human body, we have begun to lose sight of the human being.

"The gaze has shifted from the doctor's heart to the machine's eye — and in that clarity, we may have lost the warmth of being seen."

Chapter 6 – When Knowing Replaces Feeling

"In our pursuit to know everything, we forgot how to feel anything."

The monitors glowed softly in the dark clinic — heart rates, oxygen levels, diagnostic probabilities — every number precise, every metric perfect. Yet the room felt hollow. The doctor glanced at the patient, then back at the screen, unsure which deserved his attention more.

In the age of algorithmic medicine, certainty has replaced sympathy. We know more about the human body than ever before, but perhaps less about the *human being.*

This is the quiet cost of precision — the fading warmth of care in the cold light of knowledge.

The Silence of Certainty

The clinic was immaculate — white walls, sterilized air, and screens that pulsed softly with numbers that told the story of a life in perfect detail. Blood oxygen: 98%. Pulse: steady. Diagnostic confidence: 94%. Everything measurable was under control.

The doctor sat before the display, scrolling through data that left nothing unknown, nothing unseen. The machine had already rendered its judgment; the probabilities were conclusive. There was nothing more to add — except perhaps *a human presence.*

The patient sat quietly across from him, eyes searching for something that the report could not provide — a pause, a reassurance, a flicker of warmth. But the doctor's gaze, like the light from the screen, was cold and unwavering. He had all the answers, yet no words that felt adequate.

It was a perfect diagnosis in an imperfect moment — *knowledge without comfort, truth without touch.*

The Paradox of the Modern Healer

This is the paradox of modern medicine: a profession that now **knows more but feels less.** Where once the uncertainty of healing required empathy, today certainty has replaced it with efficiency. Every symptom has a code, every disease a data trail, every patient an electronic record.

But what does one heal when all the mysteries are gone? What remains of care when everything is already known?

The doctor, once an interpreter of human stories, has become an analyst of digital truths. The emotional resonance that once animated the clinical encounter has been subdued by the quiet hum of automation. The stethoscope has become symbolic — not of listening to the heart, but of verifying what the machine already knows.

And so, the new silence that fills the modern hospital is not of ignorance, but of **certainty.** A silence that feels heavier than doubt, colder than fear. It is the silence of precision without presence — a stillness where no error exists, but neither does empathy.

The New Clinical Malaise

Medicine, once a dialogue between vulnerability and compassion, now risks becoming an exchange between data and decision. The act of care — once alive with listening, touching, and understanding — is being flattened into an algorithmic routine.

The doctor, relieved of uncertainty, is burdened by detachment. The patient, surrounded by information, is starved of intimacy.

It is not ignorance but *knowing* that has begun to numb the heart of healing. In the sterile glow of predictive models and diagnostic probabilities, the soul of medicine flickers.

"When care becomes a calculation, healing loses its humanity."

This is the silence of certainty — a silence that does not arise from not knowing, but from knowing *too much* without feeling enough. And it is within this silence that the next great illness of modern medicine begins — not of the body, but of the bond between doctor and human.

The Emotional Cost of Precision

The age of automation promised to relieve doctors of burden — to make medicine faster, safer, and more precise. And in many ways, it has delivered. Diseases that once demanded hours of observation can now be flagged in seconds. Algorithms detect irregularities before the human eye can blink. Clinical dashboards organize chaos into clarity.

Yet something invisible has been lost in this perfection — something not measurable, but deeply felt. The modern physician, once a listener of suffering, has become an interpreter of numbers. The patient's pain, once described through words, gestures, and silences, now arrives as a formatted chart or a probability score.

The heartbeats are still counted, but no one listens to their rhythm anymore.

Automation and the Vanishing Conversation

Every innovation in diagnostic technology, though designed to help, quietly widens the distance between the healer and the healed. Electronic health records replace handwritten notes, predictive tools anticipate conditions before symptoms are voiced, and triage algorithms decide who is urgent before the doctor even enters the room.

These systems are marvels of logic — but they also intercept emotion. The doctor no longer begins with *"Tell me what hurts"* but with *"Let's check your results."*

What was once a conversation has become an audit. The patient, reduced to a dataset, loses not only privacy but intimacy — the feeling of being truly *seen.* And the physician, guided by precision, finds comfort in the clarity of data but alienation in its distance.

The more precise the diagnosis becomes, the less personal the experience feels.

The Data Empathy Gap

This phenomenon — the growing void between technological accuracy and emotional understanding — can be called the data empathy gap.

In this gap, the patient's suffering is translated into numerical abstraction. A person's pain becomes a waveform; their fear, a percentage; their uncertainty, a color-coded risk score. The metrics are comforting to the clinician's mind, yet strangely hollow to the patient's heart.

Empathy — once the shared ground between illness and understanding — struggles to survive in this quantified world.

Patients increasingly report feeling unheard, even when their diseases are perfectly diagnosed. It is not the medicine that fails them

— it is the *manner* of medicine. They long not for more accuracy, but for acknowledgment; not for faster results, but for human reassurance.

The data understands the disease, but not the distress.

The Hidden Toll on Physicians

This disconnection does not spare the doctors. Behind the apparent efficiency of modern clinical practice lies a quiet erosion of meaning. Physicians, once motivated by relationships and trust, now find themselves performing roles that feel mechanical — verifying, validating, approving.

Their expertise is reduced to calibration: confirming what the algorithm predicts, adjusting what the system suggests. The act of healing, once driven by presence, now feels procedural.

The emotional toll manifests as moral exhaustion — a fatigue born not from overwork but from underconnection. Many doctors describe feeling detached, even irrelevant, in a profession increasingly governed by screens and software.

Their sense of identity — once anchored in the sanctity of care — begins to dissolve in the noise of optimization. What remains is competence without closeness, accuracy without affection.

The healer, too, becomes a casualty of precision.

Reflection – When Accuracy Isolation Becomes the Norm

Data comforts the mind. It offers clarity, order, and assurance — all the things uncertainty threatens to take away. Yet in that comfort lies isolation.

Numbers create distance. They eliminate the ambiguity that often draws one human being closer to another. The spaces once filled by empathy, conversation, and doubt are now occupied by dashboards, metrics, and alerts.

In mastering disease, medicine risks losing touch with the diseased.

The precision of data comforts the mind but isolates the heart.

And in that isolation, the physician's greatest achievement — certainty — becomes their greatest sorrow.

Compassion Fatigue in Algorithmic Medicine

In earlier generations, compassion fatigue described the slow emotional wear of being exposed to too much pain. The doctor, nurse, or caregiver would reach a point of depletion — not because they didn't care, but because they cared *too much for too long.* Today, however, a quieter, stranger version of that same fatigue has emerged. In the digital clinic, the exhaustion no longer comes from *overexposure to suffering,* but from underexposure to connection.

It is a new kind of emptiness — not the pain of too much empathy, but the numbness of too little.

The New Nature of Fatigue – Emotional Depletion Without Emotion

In the age of algorithmic medicine, the physician's time is spent not beside the patient but in front of the screen. Their attention — once an act of care — has become an act of calibration. Machines now interpret most of what used to require listening, and systems flag what used to require intuition.

The result is a profession insulated from the very emotional frequencies that once sustained it. Doctors no longer burn out from *feeling too deeply* — they burn out from *not feeling at all.*

Every decision is mediated by alerts, metrics, and probabilities. The doctor trusts the device more than their instinct, because the system is faster, more accurate, and less likely to err. Yet in surrendering the emotional labor of care to automation, something essential disappears: the quiet satisfaction of presence.

A patient once said after an AI-driven consultation, *"Everything was correct, but it didn't feel like medicine."* That is the essence of this new fatigue — a form of spiritual erosion hidden beneath technological competence.

Inside the Automation Bubble

The automation bubble promises liberation — a world where machines handle the repetitive, the technical, the measurable. In theory, it should free doctors to focus on the human side of healing. In practice, it often does the opposite.

Automation creates distance disguised as efficiency. Every layer of convenience — automated notes, AI-generated prescriptions, predictive analytics — reduces the need for direct interaction. The doctor, instead of being relieved, becomes detached. They are surrounded by tools that know everything *except how it feels to care.*

The emotional circuitry of medicine — touch, empathy, reflection — is quietly bypassed in favor of streamlined workflow. What remains is performance without participation.

Efficiency may save time, but it consumes meaning.

This is the hidden cost of the automation bubble: the more friction we remove, the less fulfillment remains.

The Paradox of Distance – Productive but Empty

Emotional distance, once a coping mechanism for physicians facing intense suffering, has now become institutionalized — coded into software and system design. The distance is no longer a personal defense; it's a professional expectation.

Doctors are praised for efficiency, not empathy. Hospitals measure throughput, not trust. In this new reality, emotional suppression becomes a sign of competence.

And yet, this very detachment breeds a deeper fatigue — the fatigue of meaninglessness. A physician who sees hundreds of cases through algorithms may accomplish more, but *experience less.*

They become, as one clinician put it, *"a technician of life rather than its witness."*

This is the paradox of the modern healer:

- The less one feels, the more one produces.
- The more one produces, the less one fulfills.

Emotional distance increases productivity but decreases purpose.

Reflection – The Theft of Purpose

The machine has indeed relieved the doctor's burden — the long nights, the cognitive overload, the pressure of perfection. But in doing so, it has also quietly stolen their purpose.

For the true purpose of a physician was never merely to cure, but to *care.* To stand as a bridge between knowledge and empathy, between science and the soul. When machines take over the mechanics of knowing, what remains for the healer to hold is *feeling* — yet that too is slipping away.

In this new silence of efficiency, compassion does not scream — it simply fades.

"The machine relieves the doctor's burden, and in doing so, steals their purpose."

And thus, the doctor's greatest challenge in the algorithmic age is not mastering the machine — it is remembering how to feel in a world that rewards knowing.

The Illusion of Certainty – When Overconfidence Replaces Care

The most seductive illusion in modern medicine is certainty. For centuries, the practice of healing was shadowed by doubt — the doctor's art lay as much in managing uncertainty as in treating disease. A tremor in the hand, a hesitation in diagnosis, a quiet acknowledgment of *"I don't know yet"* — these were once signs not of weakness, but of wisdom.

But today, the language of doubt has grown obsolete. The screen rarely hesitates. The probability bar glows with confidence. And the doctor, lulled by the precision of data, begins to trust what *seems certain* more than what *feels true.*

The new mantra of the digital clinic is simple, almost devotional: "If the data says it, it must be true."

Algorithmic Precision and the Myth of Infallibility

Algorithmic systems, by design, are built to minimize uncertainty. They quantify the unquantifiable, assign probability to possibility, and turn ambiguity into clarity. Yet the precision they offer is often mistaken for perfection.

Doctors, once trained to navigate shades of gray, now live in the sharp contrast of binary outputs: malignant/benign, high/low, yes/no. Each result arrives cloaked in numerical confidence — 97%, 99%, 99.8%. But these numbers, however elegant, do not represent *truth* — they represent *likelihood.*

The danger lies not in the machine's limitations, but in our growing reverence for them. The interface of certainty, so visually reassuring, breeds quiet arrogance — not in the machine, but in the human who stops questioning it.

The physician, relieved of uncertainty, risks becoming intellectually passive. Why doubt what never doubts itself?

Cognitive Outsourcing – When the Mind Becomes Dependent

This dependency has a name: cognitive outsourcing. It is the subtle process by which human judgment yields to algorithmic confidence.

Once, the doctor's mind was a crucible of decision-making — weighing evidence, intuition, and experience. Today, much of that responsibility is delegated to systems designed to "assist." But assistance gradually becomes dependence, and dependence erodes discernment.

The clinician begins to think less and verify more. The mind adapts to convenience, not curiosity. It becomes easier — and safer — to trust the output than to challenge it.

A younger generation of doctors, raised on machine learning tools, may never experience the discomfort of doubt — and therefore, may never cultivate the humility that doubt once taught.

In surrendering uncertainty, they surrender a vital part of what made medicine human.

"The doctor's greatest risk is not being replaced by the machine, but becoming indistinguishable from it."

The Emotional Flattening of Uncertainty

Uncertainty once served as the emotional foundation of empathy. When doctors didn't know, they asked, listened, and explored. The patient's voice mattered because it was part of the mystery. The bond between them was built not on precision, but on *presence.*

Now, uncertainty is seen as inefficiency — a bug in the system, not a virtue of awareness. The hesitation that once humanized medicine has been engineered out of the process.

Where there is no doubt, there is no need to empathize. Where there is no room for surprise, there is no need to care.

This emotional flattening — the quiet disappearance of curiosity, wonder, and shared vulnerability — is perhaps the greatest unseen consequence of technological certainty. The clinic becomes quiet not because there are fewer mistakes, but because there is less conversation.

Certainty sterilizes empathy. It replaces dialogue with confirmation.

Philosophical Insight – The Comfort and Corruption of Certainty

Certainty comforts the intellect. It soothes the mind's anxiety, eliminates the tension of indecision, and replaces humility with control. But it corrupts compassion, because compassion lives in the space of unknowing — the willingness to approach another's suffering without assuming mastery over it.

The physician who never doubts cannot truly listen. The healer who never hesitates cannot truly care.

The more medicine becomes confident in its data, the more it risks losing its heart — not because knowledge is wrong, but because knowledge without wonder becomes mechanical.

Certainty comforts the intellect but corrupts compassion; it replaces curiosity with compliance.

In the end, the greatest danger of algorithmic medicine is not that machines will make mistakes, but that humans will stop caring when they don't.

The Human Element – Rediscovering Emotional Intelligence

In an era when machines have mastered diagnosis, what remains for the doctor to perfect? Not speed. Not precision. But presence. The next frontier of medicine is not computational — it is emotional.

The more the clinic fills with algorithms, the more urgently it needs *emotional intelligence* to restore its humanity.

Automation has made knowledge abundant and instant, but empathy scarce and fragile. Thus, emotional intelligence — once dismissed as a "soft skill" — now returns as the core discipline of the modern healer.

The Return of Emotional Intelligence

Emotional intelligence in medicine is not sentimentalism; it is scientific sensitivity. It means perceiving what data cannot: fear in the eyes, hesitation in the voice, the quiet panic that hides behind a patient's composure.

Machines can interpret symptoms, but not silences. They can calculate severity, but not significance.

To sense what is unsaid — that is emotional intelligence. To respond not with reassurance but with recognition — that is the new clinical artistry.

For too long, medical training prioritized intellect over intuition, competence over compassion. Yet in the sterile calm of automation, it is becoming clear that *emotion itself is information.*

Empathy is not the opposite of accuracy; it is its expansion.

Reflective Listening and the Power of Story

The rehumanization of medicine begins by reclaiming conversation. In the world of diagnostic imaging and digital dashboards, listening has become an endangered act. But it remains the most powerful diagnostic tool of all.

When doctors practice reflective listening, they don't simply hear symptoms — they uncover context. They listen *through* the words, not just *to* them. Each story reveals patterns no algorithm could infer: the social cause behind hypertension, the loneliness beneath chronic fatigue, the grief disguised as insomnia.

Narrative medicine — the practice of understanding illness through story — reawakens this dimension of care. A patient's narrative restores what data fragments: *meaning.*

Numbers reveal what the body is doing; stories reveal what the person is living. And it is in this synthesis — between data and dialogue — that medicine regains its moral center.

Empathy as Diagnostic Precision

Empathy is often mistaken for comfort — a gentle supplement to the "real" work of diagnosis. But empathy is, in fact, diagnostic precision in disguise.

An empathetic doctor perceives misalignments invisible to machines — the tone that doesn't match the words, the sudden stillness after bad news, the detail repeated twice because it still hurts to believe. These are not sentimental gestures; they are clinical data points of another kind — signals of emotional and psychological truth.

Empathy refines judgment. It shapes interpretation. It turns treatment into care.

When a physician listens with empathy, they are not just decoding pain — they are *aligning with the human pattern* beneath it. The emotional field becomes as vital to understanding as the biochemical one.

Empathy is not an alternative to logic; it is logic with awareness.

Training the Healer of the Future

The medical education of the future must therefore teach dual fluency — cognitive accuracy and emotional resonance. Students must learn to interpret ECGs and also *eyes*, to analyze data and also *doubt*, to recognize illness not only in scans but in stories.

Practical inclusion of emotional intelligence in training could mean:

- Courses in reflective dialogue, psychology, and ethics.
- Mentorship models emphasizing presence, not just performance.
- Role-playing scenarios that simulate not only emergencies but empathy.

The best future physicians will not compete with machines; they will complement them. AI will provide precision; the human will provide perspective. The synthesis of both will define what it means to heal in the 21st century.

The healer of the future will not be the one who knows the most, but the one who feels with clarity and thinks with compassion.

Reflection – Restoring the Pulse of Care

As medicine grows more intelligent, it must also grow more emotional. The human element is not nostalgia; it is necessity. Without emotional intelligence, medicine risks becoming merely the management of biological systems — efficient, accurate, and utterly hollow.

The doctor must once again become not just an analyst of disease, but a companion in recovery. Because machines may read the pulse, but only humans can restore it.

The Philosophy of Uncertainty

In a world where medicine strives for precision, uncertainty has become a heresy. Yet paradoxically, it is within uncertainty that the soul of healing resides. The machine may eliminate doubt, but the human learns *through* it — and that learning is what transforms diagnosis into care.

For centuries, uncertainty was the natural landscape of medicine. Each decision carried ambiguity; each treatment demanded courage amid the unknown. The art of healing was not to *eradicate* uncertainty, but to *navigate* it — with humility, patience, and empathy.

Now, as algorithms perfect prediction, the medical profession risks forgetting the quiet wisdom that comes from not knowing.

Uncertainty as Wisdom, Not Weakness

We tend to associate doubt with incompetence — a lack of skill or clarity. But uncertainty, when embraced consciously, becomes the birthplace of insight. It forces listening. It invites exploration. It transforms arrogance into awareness.

To say *"I don't know yet"* is not an admission of failure; it is an act of intellectual honesty and moral courage. It reminds both doctor and patient that healing is not a transaction of knowledge, but a shared journey of discovery.

Where machines operate in absolutes, humans live in nuances. And it is within those nuances — between yes and no, between cause and consequence — that compassion takes form.

"Doubt is not ignorance; it is the beginning of understanding."

The wisdom of uncertainty lies in its invitation to see patients not as problems to be solved, but as lives to be understood.

The Humility of Not Knowing

Humility is the emotional counterpart of uncertainty. The physician who accepts that they do not know everything becomes more receptive — to evidence, to experience, to emotion. They begin to see medicine not as control over life, but as cooperation *with* it.

This humility is not passivity; it is depth. It keeps curiosity alive where certainty would close it. It keeps empathy awake where confidence would numb it. In humility, the doctor stops performing as the expert and starts participating as a fellow human.

In contrast, machines cannot be humble because they cannot be aware of what they do not know. Their silence is not patience; it is absence. Their precision is not wisdom; it is calculation.

And so, the virtue that keeps medicine human — the humility of uncertainty — must remain ours alone.

"The machine eliminates doubt; the human learns from it."

Case Reflection – Presence Over Performance

Consider a scene in a modern oncology ward. A doctor sits beside a patient awaiting the results of a scan. The AI report has already arrived — predictive analytics suggest metastasis with 94% confidence. The answer is known.

Yet the doctor chooses not to read it aloud immediately.

Instead, they pause, take a seat, and listen. The patient speaks of sleepless nights, of imagining the worst, of the strange ache of waiting. The doctor listens not as a diagnostician, but as a witness.

For a few minutes, no data is interpreted, no conclusion announced. There is only presence — a shared stillness that holds space for fear, hope, and the unknown.

That moment, though medically "unproductive," is profoundly healing. Because in that pause, the doctor communicates something no algorithm can: *You are not alone in your uncertainty.*

Such acts of presence restore balance to a profession tilting dangerously toward performance. They remind us that medicine's purpose is not merely to confirm what is, but to accompany those living through what might be.

The Paradox of Knowing and Not-Knowing

To be human is to live in uncertainty; to be compassionate is to accept it. The doctor who has learned to coexist with ambiguity practices a deeper kind of science — one that unites intellect with humility.

Uncertainty, far from being an obstacle, keeps medicine ethical. It prevents arrogance, preserves empathy, and encourages collaboration. It reminds the healer that truth is never complete, that every diagnosis is a doorway, not a destination.

Machines eliminate doubt because doubt slows them down. Humans cherish doubt because doubt makes them wiser.

"The machine eliminates doubt; the human learns from it."

And therein lies the great philosophical divide of modern medicine: The machine's power lies in knowing; the human's strength lies in *understanding.*

Reflection – The Quiet Grace of Doubt

When healing becomes certain, it becomes mechanical. When it allows space for uncertainty, it becomes sacred.

Every act of care requires a measure of surrender — a willingness to sit within the limits of knowledge and still offer presence, kindness, and hope. That is not inefficiency; it is integrity.

In the age of perfect data, we must remember that the imperfect silence between questions often heals more than the most confident answer.

To doubt wisely is to care deeply.

For in the space where certainty ends, humanity begins.

Reflection – The Loss and the Lesson

The story of modern medicine is often told as a triumph of intelligence — from ignorance to insight, from intuition to information. We built machines that could see what we could not, predict what we could never guess, and measure what we could only feel. Yet in the pursuit of knowing everything, we quietly began to forget how to feel anything.

This is not a failure of technology; it is a consequence of imbalance — an overgrowth of intellect without the nourishment of emotion. Algorithmic medicine has given us precision, but it has taken something equally vital in return: *the texture of care, the warmth of understanding, the grace of doubt.*

We gained mastery over uncertainty but lost the meaning that uncertainty once carried.

The Emotional and Ethical Cost of Algorithmic Knowing

The emotional cost of our technological ascent is subtle yet devastating. Doctors are no longer exhausted by the weight of compassion but by its absence. They no longer break down under the pain of caring too deeply, but under the emptiness of not caring enough.

The patient, meanwhile, feels more seen and less understood than ever before. The data knows their biology, but not their biography. The system tracks every beat of their heart, yet not the tremor of their fear.

In this transformation, medicine has become informationally omniscient and emotionally impoverished.

The ethical cost follows close behind. When certainty replaces empathy, decision-making becomes efficient but morally shallow. A perfect diagnosis delivered without compassion may save a body but wound a soul. The duty to heal is fulfilled, but the act of healing is diminished.

Precision without feeling may preserve life, but it cannot restore living.

Medicine's new dilemma: the body survives, the person disappears.

The New Moral Imperative – Restoring Feeling to Knowledge

The lesson of this era is not to resist technology, but to reclaim humanity within it. The moral challenge of the 21st-century physician is not to outthink the machine, but to *outfeel* it.

The framework of medicine must expand — from knowledge as accumulation to knowledge as connection. Data alone cannot guide care; it must be infused with awareness, humility, and compassion. We must build systems not only to see more clearly, but to *care more deeply.*

This is the new Hippocratic oath: To heal with precision, but to understand with presence. To use intelligence as a tool, not a barrier, between souls.

For medicine was never meant to be about the triumph of intellect over suffering; it was meant to be the meeting point of both.

The future of medicine lies not in artificial intelligence, but in augmented empathy.

Dual Truth – Precision Saves Lives, Compassion Saves Meanings

There are two truths in healing, both essential and eternal. Precision saves lives. It prevents error, eliminates guesswork, and brings light to the darkest recesses of the body. Compassion saves meanings. It turns survival into living, treatment into understanding, and care into connection.

To prioritize one over the other is to fragment the human experience of healing. A surgeon can remove a tumor with flawless accuracy, but only empathy can help a patient make peace with the scar. An AI can predict depression, but only another human can sit beside someone who feels it.

Medicine's future depends not on choosing between the two truths but on weaving them together — to create a science of care that is both brilliant and kind.

The hand must know what the heart understands.

The Lesson Hidden in the Loss

Every loss carries a lesson, and this one is simple yet profound: The more we mechanize care, the more deliberately we must humanize it. The more we automate diagnosis, the more intentionally we must preserve presence.

We once defined progress as replacing the uncertain doctor with the perfect machine. Now we must redefine it as *teaching the perfect machine to serve the imperfect human.*

The doctor of tomorrow will stand between two intelligences — one that calculates and one that feels — and their greatness will depend on how gracefully they can unite the two.

"We learned to know everything, except how it feels to be known."

Closing Reflection – The Silent Wisdom of Balance

Perhaps this is the real lesson of algorithmic medicine: not that we have lost our humanity, but that we are finally beginning to notice its absence. Technology has completed its part of the evolution — it has given us the power to know. Now, it is our turn to evolve — to remember how to *understand.*

Knowledge makes us accurate. Awareness makes us wise. Compassion makes us human.

And in that delicate balance between the precision of intelligence and the imperfection of empathy, healing will once again find its voice.

"Error as Enlightenment"

Medicine, in its relentless pursuit of perfection, has reached a strange kind of silence — one filled not with ignorance, but with confidence so complete that it leaves no room for humility. We have built systems that almost never falter, predictions that rarely fail, and processes that leave little to question. Yet in this perfection, something essential has been muted: the *human capacity to learn through mistakes.*

Error, once the teacher of wisdom, has been exiled from the clinical imagination.

And yet, perhaps that exile is premature.

The Forgotten Teacher: Error

Throughout history, human progress has been written in the ink of mistakes. Every discovery, from vaccines to antibiotics to surgical innovation, was born not from certainty, but from missteps — from accidents that revealed what intention could not. In this sense, error has never been the enemy of truth; it has been its most honest mirror.

But as medicine becomes algorithmic, it grows increasingly allergic to error. Machines are designed to minimize deviation; humans are trained to fear it. We now inhabit an ecosystem of precision where mistakes are not merely corrected — they are *erased.*

Yet what happens to growth when error disappears? What happens to empathy when nothing is left to forgive?

When doctors no longer err, they no longer experience the humility that gives meaning to healing. When algorithms fail, we rush to fix the code — but seldom pause to ask *why the failure mattered.*

There is a deeper truth hidden here: every error, whether human or mechanical, contains insight about the limits of perception.

The Coming Reflection – Error as Enlightenment

The next chapter, *"Error as Enlightenment,"* turns toward this paradox — that imperfection may be medicine's last remaining source of wisdom. It explores how both human fallibility and machine malfunction reveal something larger than technical failure: they expose the boundaries of understanding, the fragility of knowledge, and the enduring necessity of doubt.

It asks:

- Can we find meaning in mistakes, rather than shame?
- Can failure become feedback — not for correction alone, but for comprehension?
- And can machines, in their errors, remind us of what it means to be human — to strive, to misjudge, to learn, to evolve?

For in the end, perfection may produce efficiency, but imperfection produces *insight.* The flaw is not a weakness of design — it is the signature of consciousness.

Closing Reflection

As this chapter ends, we stand at the threshold of a new moral understanding: that both man and machine must fail to truly know themselves. The precision we have built has given us mastery, but it has taken away mystery. It has given us answers, but it has silenced our wonder.

If the previous chapter revealed the emotional cost of certainty, the next will reveal the *spiritual value of error.*

"Perfection silenced our empathy; perhaps imperfection will teach us to listen again."

Chapter 7 – Error as Enlightenment

"Perfection builds machines; mistakes build meaning."

The diagnosis was wrong. The screen declared *"malignant"* — 96% probability. The patient's world collapsed in seconds. But a week later, the biopsy returned negative. Relief flooded the room, yet beneath it lingered something deeper — a question that data could not answer.

The machine had failed, but in that failure, everyone began to see differently. The doctor re-examined the scan, noticing subtleties the algorithm had overlooked. The engineers revised their dataset, discovering hidden bias. The patient, once frightened by the machine's authority, learned that even the most advanced intelligence could still *misunderstand the body.*

That single mistake became a quiet teacher — reminding all that truth, in medicine, does not live in certainty, but in correction.

We often fear error as the end of knowledge, when in fact, it is where knowledge begins.

The Wisdom Hidden in Mistakes

The day began with quiet confidence. The new AI diagnostic system had been running flawlessly for weeks — analyzing scans, flagging anomalies, and delivering reports faster than any human team ever could. Then, it happened.

The screen flashed a red warning: "Malignant lesion detected — 98% probability." The patient froze. The nurse whispered. The doctor, momentarily trusting the machine's conviction, scheduled an urgent biopsy. For forty-eight hours, fear ruled the room.

When the results came back, the tumor was benign. The machine was wrong — or so it seemed.

But when the radiologist revisited the scan, he saw something the algorithm had been trying, in its strange statistical way, to signal. The growth was benign today, yes — but its cellular structure hinted at a mutation trend that might one day turn dangerous. The doctor had missed that subtle trajectory; the AI had over-interpreted it. Each had seen half the truth.

What emerged from this moment was not blame, but awareness. The error became an educator.

Error as Mirror, Not Mistake

In that small event lay the larger story of our time — a quiet revolution in how we define knowledge itself. For centuries, medicine treated mistakes as failures to be erased, punished, or forgotten. But now, in the age of algorithms, each error leaves a digital footprint — a precise map of where human judgment and machine logic diverge.

Every misclassification, every false alarm, every overlooked anomaly is no longer a dead end; it is a reflection of how perception works — and where it fails. Error, in this new world, is not the enemy of truth but its most honest companion.

We learn not because we are flawless, but because we are corrigible.

The Doctor and the Machine – Two Ways of Seeing

When the radiologist re-examined the case, he realized something profound: he and the machine had not disagreed — they had completed each other.

The AI, unburdened by fatigue or emotion, saw the statistical rhythm of pixels — the probability of change. The human, shaped by experience and empathy, saw the person behind the scan — the story, the fear, the consequence.

Neither was wrong; both were incomplete.

Together, they formed a fuller truth — one built not on certainty, but on mutual correction.

The lesson was clear: error had become the new teacher of wisdom, the bridge between two forms of intelligence — one biological, one digital.

Philosophical Premise – The Paradox of Perfection

Perfection is efficient, but sterile. Error is disruptive, but alive.

Perfection closes the loop of learning; error keeps it open. Perfection brings precision; error brings perspective. Perfection makes machines; error makes meaning.

When everything works as expected, nothing new is discovered. When something fails, reality reveals another layer of itself — the hidden variables, the unspoken assumptions, the blind spots of both silicon and soul.

The doctor's humility and the algorithm's misfire together created what pure accuracy never could: understanding.

Reflection: "Perfection reveals efficiency, but error reveals understanding. For in every mistake lies a mirror — not of failure, but of truth unfinished."

The Machine's Fallibility – When AI Misdiagnoses

The promise of Artificial Intelligence in medicine has always carried an unspoken assumption — that machines, unlike humans, do not err. They do not tire, they do not panic, they do not overlook. They do not have moods, biases, or blind spots. They process data, and data does not lie.

At least, that's what we wanted to believe.

But soon after the first wave of clinical AI deployments, the illusion began to fracture. The "digital doctor" turned out to have its own form of blindness — subtler, statistical, and far less visible.

False Positives, False Promises

In 2019, a deep-learning system trained to detect lung nodules in chest X-rays achieved near-perfect accuracy — until it was tested on data from a different hospital. Suddenly, its performance collapsed. Why? Because it had learned to recognize the scanner's watermark, not the tumor. The machine had confused the *signature of the device* with the *signature of disease.*

In dermatology, AI systems trained on light-skinned populations began over-diagnosing melanoma in darker skin tones. The error wasn't technical — it was sociological. The machine reflected a human oversight — the absence of diversity in its training data.

And in radiology, triage systems meant to detect brain hemorrhages sometimes raised false alarms when encountering metallic implants or rare anatomical variations. What humans dismissed as artifact, the algorithm read as injury.

Each case was a reminder: the machine does not understand what it sees — it only repeats what it has been taught.

The Myth of Mechanical Infallibility

AI is often perceived as incorruptible — an objective mind above human prejudice. But every algorithm carries the fingerprints of its maker. Behind every model lies a thousand small decisions — which data to include, which variables to weigh, which anomalies to ignore.

These invisible human choices shape the machine's sense of reality. And when the model fails, it does so not because it *broke*, but because it *faithfully mirrored our own imperfection.*

AI does not make errors in spite of its design — it makes them *because* of it.

It is, in essence, an amplifier of human limitation. It reproduces not only intelligence but also ignorance — at scale.

The more data we give it, the more confident it becomes; the more confident it becomes, the less we question it. This is how errors evolve from isolated glitches into systemic illusions — invisible yet powerful.

The Error Loop – How Bias Multiplies

In medicine, small biases can ripple into catastrophic consequences.

A dataset over-representing one demographic can skew risk models for others. A mislabeled scan can teach an entire system to misinterpret similar cases. A poorly calibrated algorithm can prioritize false positives, leading to unnecessary biopsies, anxiety, and expense.

Once deployed, these biases feed back into the system — every misdiagnosis creates new data, which the model learns from again, reinforcing its own distortion. Thus emerges the *error loop* — a cycle where bias creates output, output becomes data, and data revalidates bias.

The result: a self-fulfilling prophecy of precision.

The system grows increasingly confident — and increasingly wrong.

Calculation vs. Comprehension

Every time a machine misdiagnoses, it reveals the boundary of its intelligence — the difference between calculation and comprehension.

A neural network can identify millions of patterns in seconds, but it cannot *know* what a tumor means to a life, a family, or a fear. It can detect, classify, and predict — but it cannot interpret. It lacks not knowledge, but *context.*

Human comprehension, in contrast, is born of imperfection. We learn not only from what is correct but from what hurts, surprises, and confuses us. Machines optimize; humans *understand.*

And so every mechanical mistake is an invitation — not to abandon technology, but to reinsert humanity into it.

Reflection – The Human Return

The AI's misdiagnosis is not the end of truth; it is the reopening of it. Each error is a message — not of failure, but of humility. It whispers: *You are still needed here.*

Machines can map probability, but not meaning. They can locate the illness, but not the suffering. They can predict the future, but not prepare the heart.

Every misstep of an algorithm is an opportunity for doctors to rediscover their role — not as technicians verifying output, but as interpreters of consequence.

For in that fragile space where the machine falters, medicine breathes again — not as code, but as care.

Philosophical Insight: *Each machine error exposes the boundary between calculation and comprehension — a reminder that perfection without awareness is blindness, repeated at scale.*

Human Fallibility – The Strength of Intuitive Error

In the grand theater of medicine, human error has always played the role of both villain and teacher. It kills, but it also evolves. It humbles, but it also illumines.

Where machines err through blind calculation, humans err through *feeling stretched beyond reason.* A physician's mistake often arises not from ignorance, but from the friction between intuition and intellect — from caring too much, from believing too deeply, from hoping where statistics have already given up.

And therein lies a paradox: the same emotional currents that sometimes cloud human judgment are also the very forces that propel human discovery.

The Anatomy of Human Error

Every clinician knows the weight of fallibility. A missed sign, a delayed test, a misplaced assumption — each one burns itself into memory. But unlike machine failure, human error has depth. It is rarely random; it carries intent, context, emotion.

A surgeon's trembling hand after 16 hours of operating. A general practitioner's quick diagnosis based on the faint echo of past cases. A pediatrician's decision to wait and observe, guided not by protocol, but by a mother's anxiety.

These are not errors born of negligence — they are *errors of empathy,* the byproducts of being human in an imperfect world.

The Evolutionary Power of Being Wrong

Humanity's progress — in medicine, science, and philosophy — has never followed a straight line of certainty. It has moved in spirals of error, reflection, and realization.

Penicillin was discovered because Alexander Fleming left a petri dish unattended — a *mistake* that changed history. The discovery of X-rays came from Wilhelm Röntgen's curiosity about a mysterious glow — a *side effect* no calculation predicted. And many diagnostic protocols were rewritten not because of planned success, but because of *unexpected failure.*

Each wrong turn created the conditions for deeper understanding.

Error, in this sense, is not a defect in the human system — it is its engine. It forces adaptation. It demands humility. It transforms learning from memorization into metamorphosis.

Machines improve by correction; humans evolve by reflection.

The Intuitive Edge – The Gift Hidden in Mistakes

Unlike algorithms, the human brain operates with layers of *uncertainty tolerance.* We can act without complete information. We can intuit, guess, empathize, and imagine — all risky, error-prone processes that paradoxically allow innovation.

When a doctor makes a mistake, they don't just revise the data; they re-examine their perception. They learn not only what went wrong, but *why they thought it was right.*

This recursive self-awareness — the ability to confront one's own fallibility — is the birthplace of wisdom. Machines have feedback; humans have conscience. Machines can adjust; humans can transform.

The Strength of the Fallible Mind

The human mind errs because it *feels.* It reacts to pressure, compassion, fear, and love — those immeasurable forces that shape perception far beyond data. It is not precision that defines human intelligence, but resilience — the ability to recover, reinterpret, and realign after every failure.

To be fallible is not to be flawed; it is to be *alive.* Perfection stagnates; fallibility flows. A doctor who never doubts cannot heal beyond protocol; a system that never fails cannot learn beyond code.

Philosophical Reflection: "The human mind errs because it feels; the machine errs because it cannot. One stumbles toward meaning, the other circles precision — but only the one that bleeds can truly evolve."

The Dialogue Between Errors – Man and Machine Learning Each Other

For most of history, the relationship between human and machine was defined by command — one giving orders, the other executing them. But in the age of Doctor AI, that hierarchy is dissolving. The machine no longer merely obeys; it *interprets.* And the human no longer merely decides; they *collaborate.*

Yet this partnership does not evolve through perfection — it matures through mutual fallibility. The most meaningful progress between man and machine now happens not when they are both right, but when they are wrong in different ways.

Collaborative Fallibility – A New Model of Learning

In traditional medicine, error was individual — a doctor's oversight, a misjudged symptom, a missed correlation. In algorithmic medicine, error becomes relational — a conversation between two intelligences, each illuminating the other's blind spots.

This is *collaborative fallibility* — the process by which human intuition and machine logic, through their respective missteps, gradually converge toward wisdom neither could reach alone.

When the machine errs, it exposes the limits of data. When the human errs, it exposes the limits of experience. Together, they chart the boundary of knowledge.

Case Illustration – The Learning Loop

A radiologist reviews a chest CT. The AI flags a small nodule in the left lung as malignant. The human disagrees — experience tells her it's likely a benign scar. She dismisses the alert, adds a note, and finalizes the report.

Weeks later, a follow-up scan confirms the AI was right. She corrects her notes, uploads the findings, and the AI system retrains — adjusting its detection pattern based on this new ground truth.

Months later, in a different case, the same AI flags another subtle lesion — one the doctor nearly overlooks. This time, she pauses. The machine's earlier "mistake" has refined her judgment; her earlier "correction" has refined its model.

They have, in essence, *taught each other to see more completely.*

What once was an error became a dialogue — and the dialogue became the architecture of deeper accuracy.

Error as the Connective Tissue of Progress

In this co-evolutionary process, error becomes the connective tissue of healing itself. Every false alarm teaches restraint. Every missed diagnosis teaches attention. Every disagreement between human and machine adds a new layer of shared insight.

Just as the immune system learns through exposure, the medical ecosystem learns through misalignment. Mistakes are no longer the fractures of knowledge — they are its joints, allowing the body of science to move, flex, and grow.

Each correction, each iteration, each act of humility redefines the relationship — transforming medicine from a discipline of authority into a dialogue of awareness.

Mutual Learning – The Birth of Hybrid Wisdom

When the physician and the algorithm learn from each other's errors, something extraordinary happens: They begin to form a hybrid intelligence — a living synthesis of logic and empathy, data and doubt.

The machine lends speed, consistency, and depth; the human contributes meaning, emotion, and ethical direction. Neither is complete alone — one sees patterns, the other perceives purpose.

Through reciprocal imperfection, they construct something that transcends both: wisdom through alignment.

Not the perfection of code, nor the intuition of instinct — but a new, shared awareness that accepts error as the foundation of truth.

Reflection: "Medicine advances not through being right, but through learning why it was wrong. In every mutual mistake, man and machine recognize each other — not as rivals of intelligence, but as partners in awakening."

Misalignment as the Mirror of Consequence

No mistake exists in isolation. Every error — human or machine — casts ripples far beyond the moment of its occurrence. A misdiagnosis is not simply a wrong answer; it is a mirror that reflects the deeper alignments and misalignments within the entire ecosystem of intelligence — data, decision, and duty.

The failure itself is only the surface symptom. The *consequences* that follow — the reactions, reflections, and reforms it provokes — become the real source of wisdom.

Error teaches accuracy; misalignment teaches awareness.

Misalignment as the True Teacher

When an AI system misses a rare condition, the immediate concern is correction — update the data, retrain the model, fix the bug. But beneath the surface lies a subtler question: *Why did the system fail in the first place?*

Perhaps the training data lacked diversity. Perhaps the human oversight was rushed. Perhaps the machine's confidence score was over-weighted. Or perhaps, more deeply, the purpose of diagnosis was reduced to detection alone — detached from care, empathy, or context.

Misalignment reveals not just where logic broke, but where intelligence lost its coherence with meaning. It is not the failure of performance; it is the failure of purpose.

Each misstep therefore becomes a teacher of consequence — not only highlighting what went wrong, but why it mattered.

Consequence Intelligence – Learning from the Aftermath

In the philosophy of Consequence Intelligence — a cornerstone of both ethical AI and Universal Energy Dynamics (UED) thought — every ripple of error triggers self-correction through awareness of its impact.

Human or machine, intelligence matures not through success but through encountering consequence.

A delayed diagnosis, for instance, is not just a technical lapse. It initiates a moral chain reaction:

- The doctor reflects on missed signs and the cost of overconfidence.
- The hospital reviews workflow and accountability.
- The AI engineers examine the dataset for hidden bias.
- The patient's story enters medical ethics discussions, reshaping policy.

Out of a single misalignment, an entire web of awareness unfolds — one that deepens responsibility at every level.

In this way, error becomes the field through which conscience evolves. It refines systems, softens egos, and demands humility from all forms of intelligence — organic or synthetic.

The Ripple of Realization – How Error Reshapes the System

Every consequence births a response, and every response, when acknowledged, leads to re-alignment. This is the moral physics of medicine — the ripple logic of growth.

A delayed cancer detection results in new triage protocols. A false negative in a rural clinic inspires an audit on data diversity. A patient complaint sparks a movement for transparency in AI-driven diagnostics.

In each case, consequence becomes curriculum. It redefines intelligence as participation in correction, not just computation of results.

Machines retrain their models; humans retrain their morality. Together, they create an ecosystem where wisdom is the residue of consequence understood.

Philosophy – The Real Curriculum of Intelligence

Perfection teaches nothing; it leaves no trace, no reason to think, no need to grow. But consequence — that gentle, sometimes brutal feedback of reality — teaches everything.

It tells the human: "You are not infallible; act with empathy." It tells the machine: "You are not omniscient; adapt to diversity." It tells both: "Awareness, not accuracy, defines intelligence."

True intelligence — whether biological or artificial — is not the capacity to avoid error, but the grace to evolve through it.

In this light, misalignment becomes sacred. It is the space where logic meets humility, where progress meets patience, where understanding begins to breathe.

Reflection: "Consequence is the curriculum of consciousness. Machines learn correction; humans learn compassion. Together they learn the one truth that endures — that misalignment is not failure, but the mirror through which all intelligence sees itself."

The Philosophy of Forgiveness in Medicine

Forgiveness, in its deepest sense, is not about moral absolution — it is about *understanding complexity*. In medicine, where every decision can mean the difference between life and death, forgiveness feels almost scandalous. How can one forgive a misdiagnosis? A delayed reaction? A flawed algorithm that cost someone time, pain, or trust?

Yet without forgiveness — without the ability to look at failure through the lens of comprehension rather than condemnation — medicine itself would cease to evolve.

Because every advance in healing begins with one courageous act: the willingness to learn from what went wrong.

Forgiveness as Epistemic Humility

Forgiveness, when stripped of its moral weight, becomes a form of epistemic humility — the recognition that all knowledge, no matter how sophisticated, is incomplete.

Doctors err because medicine is not omniscient. Machines err because data is not infinite. Patients suffer because life itself resists total understanding.

To forgive, then, is to acknowledge the limitations of knowing — to admit that awareness grows only by confronting its own boundaries.

Forgiveness is not saying, "It's okay you failed." It is saying, "Failure has meaning." It transforms error from a wound into a window — a way to see the deeper laws of consequence at play.

"Forgiveness is the humility of intelligence — the awareness that truth, like healing, is never finished."

Human Error and the Weight of Accountability

When a physician makes a mistake, the moral instinct is to assign blame. Accountability is necessary, of course, but beyond punishment lies something more profound: reflection.

A doctor who hides behind excuses learns nothing; a doctor who faces their error with honesty begins to evolve. Every error reopens the dialogue between judgment and empathy, reminding the healer that they are still human — and that humanity, not perfection, is the core of healing itself.

The strength of the medical profession has never been its infallibility; it has been its capacity to recover from error with compassion.

True accountability is not the absence of forgiveness — it is forgiveness practiced through action, reform, and renewed intention.

Machine Error and the Demand for Interpretation

When an algorithm errs, we cannot scold it or shame it — it feels neither guilt nor remorse. But that absence of emotion does not absolve us of ethical responsibility. Instead, it calls for something uniquely human: interpretation.

Forgiving machine error means refusing to see it as failure alone. It is an invitation to look beyond the malfunction — to understand *why* it happened and *what* it reveals about the system that produced it.

The act of interpreting algorithmic mistakes is, in essence, an act of compassion — not toward the machine, but toward the collective intelligence it represents.

Forgiveness, in this context, becomes a scientific virtue: it transforms blame into curiosity, and curiosity into progress.

The Shared Humility of Imperfection

Both man and machine are bound by imperfection — one emotional, the other computational. But humility unites them.

When a physician forgives themselves, they create space to think clearly again. When engineers forgive a system's failure, they create space for innovation. When institutions forgive collectively — not to forget, but to understand — they nurture ethical progress.

Forgiveness is the bridge between error and evolution. It keeps the moral field of medicine alive, flexible, and capable of growth.

Without forgiveness, every mistake becomes a scar; with it, every mistake becomes a seed.

Reflection – Forgiving to Understand

The act of forgiving error — whether human or artificial — is also the act of acknowledging complexity. It says: "This went wrong because reality is intricate, because intelligence is layered, because consequence is real."

In forgiving, we do not excuse. We *expand.* We make room for the multiple truths that coexist in every decision, every diagnosis, every human attempt to control uncertainty.

Philosophical Reflection: "Forgiveness is not the end of justice; it is the beginning of understanding. For every error we forgive, we widen the horizon of what intelligence can see."

Closing Insight

Medicine without forgiveness would be a field of fear — one where every mistake is punished and every learner silenced. But with forgiveness, medicine becomes what it was always meant to be: a living dialogue between knowledge and compassion.

Machines may never know remorse, but humans can feel it — and in feeling it, they ensure that progress never loses its conscience.

"To forgive an error is to honor the truth it tried to reveal."

Reflection – Error as Illumination

In the ancient practice of alchemy, the transformation of base metal into gold was never truly about chemistry — it was about awareness. The alchemists knew that transformation begins where failure refuses to be wasted.

Modern medicine, guided now by algorithms and intelligence, stands in the same place. Its real evolution will not come from eradicating error but from learning how to see through it.

Error is no longer a shadow to be feared — it is the light that outlines the limits of our vision.

Error as Mirror

Every mistake — whether born of human intuition or machine calculation — is a mirror reflecting the boundary between what we know and what we think we know. When a diagnosis goes wrong, it shows not just a lapse in method, but a distortion in perception — a reminder that truth is never absolute, only contextual.

Human errors mirror emotional overreach, fatigue, or misplaced certainty. Machine errors mirror blind data, missing context, and mechanical overconfidence.

Each reflection reveals a facet of our collective blindness, and in recognizing it, we begin to see *more honestly.*

The mirror of error, therefore, is not cruel — it is compassionate. It returns to us the humbling reminder that every act of knowing must begin with the awareness of not knowing.

Error as Bridge

Between the physician and the algorithm lies a vast and delicate bridge — built not of code or compassion, but of *correction.*

Each time man and machine disagree, that bridge strengthens. Each mutual mistake creates a dialogue that makes both sides wiser.

The machine learns the nuance of human exception; the doctor learns the precision of machine patterning. Through this iterative humility, a new intelligence takes form — a hybrid wisdom, born from the cross-pollination of fallibility.

Error, then, is not a crack in the bridge of progress — it is the bridge itself.

Without it, there is no connection between experience and evidence, intuition and information, empathy and efficiency.

Error as Teacher

No teacher is more honest than failure. Where success flatters, error instructs. It removes illusion, exposes arrogance, and demands reflection.

Medicine, more than any other human endeavor, has evolved through such lessons. Every procedural refinement, every breakthrough drug, every ethical reform — all born from something once misjudged, misread, or misunderstood.

A century of scientific progress is, at its heart, a chronicle of refined mistakes.

"We grow not by being right, but by realizing what being wrong reveals."

Error teaches the most difficult virtue in both humans and machines — humility. And humility, in turn, becomes the soil where awareness blooms.

Transforming Mistake into Meaning

The future of medicine will not belong to those who design flawless systems, but to those who can interpret imperfection meaningfully.

Every error, when observed consciously, becomes a data point of wisdom. A delayed diagnosis becomes a policy improvement. A misprediction becomes a deeper model. A misunderstanding between doctor and patient becomes a lesson in communication.

When seen in this way, failure ceases to be a flaw — it becomes *feedback*. It transforms punishment into progress, guilt into growth, and precision into understanding.

Error as Illumination

Error, in its truest form, is not darkness — it is light scattered across the edges of awareness. It is the flash that reveals where our comprehension ends and reality begins.

To eliminate all error would be to eliminate learning itself — to strip medicine of its humanity and AI of its evolution.

Error is the friction that keeps intelligence alive, the necessary resistance that turns raw data into wisdom.

In its shimmer lies the most profound truth: We err, therefore we learn. We fail, therefore we see. We stumble, therefore we become aware.

"Error is not the absence of knowledge, but the presence of awareness."

Closing Reflection – The Light Within the Flaw

The world once feared error as the opposite of order. Now, we begin to see it as the *heartbeat of learning itself.* The machine, through its miscalculations, discovers the edges of precision. The human, through their misjudgments, discovers the depth of perception.

Together, they remind us that perfection is sterile — only imperfection grows.

To err is not merely human; it is intelligent. To learn from it — that is wisdom illuminated.

"The Observer's Burden"

Every mistake leaves behind a residue — not just in data, but in consciousness. Once we begin to learn from error, we also begin to see differently. What was once dismissed as failure becomes feedback; what was once unseen now demands awareness.

But awareness carries a price. For in a world where every act of seeing generates new data, to observe is no longer neutral — it is consequential.

Medicine has now entered a new moral terrain.

From Error to Observation – The Next Evolution

If *error* taught us humility, *observation* will test our integrity. When AI systems record, analyze, and predict every fragment of biological and behavioral data, observation itself becomes an act of power.

The physician's gaze once diagnosed; now it defines reality. The algorithm's gaze once detected; now it determines action.

Each observation influences the patient's course of treatment, their anxiety, their faith in recovery — even their perception of self. To look is to alter. To measure is to decide. To record is to define.

This is the new paradox of Doctor AI: The more precisely we observe, the more profoundly we interfere.

Observation is no longer passive; it shapes consequence. And with consequence comes responsibility.

Observation as Ethical Act

When every image becomes a data point, and every heartbeat a prediction, the act of "seeing" becomes a moral choice.

What do we choose to notice? What do we choose to ignore? Whose pain gets documented, and whose remains invisible?

The human observer, once seen as a neutral instrument of diagnosis, now stands at the intersection of technology, ethics, and existence.

Every scan, every sensor, every algorithmic gaze adds to the expanding archive of human life — and each observation silently rewrites the patient's reality.

To observe, then, is to participate in creation itself — to alter what is seen by the very act of seeing.

The observer, whether human or artificial, carries a burden — the duty to see responsibly, with awareness of consequence.

From Learning to Accountability

The journey from error to observation marks the shift from awareness to accountability. If error teaches us where truth hides, observation demands that we decide what to *do* with that truth.

It is no longer enough to understand how AI learns — we must now question how it watches. It is no longer enough for humans to correct machines — we must now co-govern their gaze.

The next frontier of technophilosophy in medicine is not about smarter diagnosis, but about conscious seeing. The observer's role has expanded — from witnessing life to shaping it.

Closing Reflection

As we step from the realm of error into the realm of observation, the challenge deepens. The problem is no longer *Can we see clearly?* but *Can we see responsibly?*

Every lens, every sensor, every doctor, and every algorithm becomes part of a shared moral vision — one where perception itself must be ethical.

"Error showed us where truth hides; now observation will show us what truth demands."

Chapter 8 – The Observer's Burden

"To see is no longer to witness — it is to intervene."

The doctor hovers over the screen, cursor trembling above the final click. The AI has flagged the scan with a 92% probability of malignancy. The patient waits outside, unaware that a single confirmation will decide not only the treatment plan, but the story their life will now tell.

In that moment, the act of *seeing* becomes an act of *creation.* Once the diagnosis is recorded, the possibilities collapse — uncertainty gives way to certainty, and the patient's reality changes forever.

Observation, once thought to be neutral, now carries the weight of consequence. The more medicine learns to see, the more it must answer for how it sees.

In the age of Doctor AI, the observer is no longer a bystander to truth — the observer has become its architect.

The Gaze That Changes the Game

The radiologist sat before the glowing monitor, the room dim except for the quiet hum of machines. On the screen, a CT scan of a patient's chest awaited her final verdict. The AI algorithm had already flagged a region of interest — *"malignancy likelihood: 87%."* The data was clean, the margins sharp, the metrics confident. All she had to do was click "Confirm Diagnosis."

Her finger hovered over the mouse, suspended between knowing and deciding. That single click would trigger a cascade: treatment authorization, insurance notification, surgery scheduling, emotional devastation — or relief. One click would turn probability into destiny.

In that instant, she was not just *reading* an image; she was *collapsing reality.*

Observation as Creation

In that small gesture — the motion of a human hand over a digital button — the ancient role of the observer transformed. What once was an act of noticing had become an act of creation. Before the click, the patient existed in a cloud of probabilities — maybe sick, maybe well. After the click, only one reality remained.

This is the paradox at the heart of modern medicine: the gaze that diagnoses also defines.

Just as in quantum physics, where observation determines the state of a particle, in data-driven medicine the act of observation determines the state of the person. A measurement, once taken, alters the system that produced it. A diagnosis, once made, alters the life it describes.

In both worlds, there is no longer such a thing as neutral observation — because to see is to intervene.

The Quantum Parallel – Medicine's New Physics of Truth

In the quantum world, a particle exists in multiple states until observed; the moment it is measured, the wave collapses into a definite outcome. In medicine, something eerily similar happens every day.

A test result, an image scan, a risk score — each observation narrows infinite biological uncertainty into a single label. "Cancer." "Normal." "Abnormal." "Inconclusive." The patient's universe, once open with possibility, constricts into the certainty of a medical definition.

The irony is that even this so-called "certainty" is an illusion — a construct of the observer's framework. The diagnosis depends on thresholds chosen by human committees, algorithms trained on selective data, and interpretations influenced by context and bias.

Yet to the patient, the label becomes absolute truth. The observer's perception has materialized reality.

The Ethical Tension – When Seeing Becomes Deciding

In the analog age, the physician's gaze was personal and interpretive — an encounter between two living beings. Today, that gaze is amplified by systems that see deeper, faster, and wider than the human eye ever could. But with that amplification comes an escalation of consequence.

Every time an AI system highlights an anomaly, every time a clinician validates its judgment, a decision is made — one that will ripple through the patient's body, emotions, finances, and identity.

Observation has become decision disguised as vision. The act of looking is now inseparable from the act of choosing.

The modern medical observer holds the power not just to detect disease, but to define the boundaries of health, normalcy, and hope. Each gaze, amplified by code and data, carries moral weight.

Philosophical Premise – No Neutral Gaze Remains

The myth of objectivity is collapsing. There is no view from nowhere — not in physics, not in medicine, not in intelligence. Every act of seeing involves participation.

When we observe, we alter. When we measure, we define. When we interpret, we create.

Doctor AI, in this light, is not merely a diagnostic tool; it is a new kind of observer — one whose perception rewrites reality at scale. And yet, it still depends on human participation to give that reality *meaning.*

The physician is no longer just an analyst of data but a co-creator of truth — sharing responsibility with the machine for every world they bring into being.

Reflection: "In the age of data-driven medicine, to see is to decide. Every observation reshapes reality, and every click of confirmation writes a new truth. The gaze no longer reports — it creates."

The Quantum Parallel – When Observation Creates Reality

In physics, the observer effect is a quiet revolution — the recognition that to measure something is to change it. When a scientist observes an electron, the act of measurement collapses its wave of probabilities into a single, defined state. The observer is no longer external; their very act of watching alters the outcome.

Reality, in the quantum world, is not a fixed script but a dynamic unfolding — shaped by the act of perception itself. Nowhere, perhaps, is this principle more vividly mirrored than in modern medicine.

For in medicine, too, observation creates reality.

Medicine and the Quantum Gaze

When a patient enters a hospital, they are not just examined — they are *transformed by being observed.*

The diagnostic gaze, whether human or algorithmic, does more than record data; it defines the person it sees. Before the test, the patient exists in a field of uncertainty: perhaps healthy, perhaps not. After the test, that uncertainty collapses into a single identity — "normal," "abnormal," "at risk," "positive," or "negative."

In that moment, a human being becomes a category. The body becomes data. And the gaze that sees them becomes part of the story of who they are.

Medicine's observer effect is not metaphorical — it is profoundly real. Every measurement changes the patient's biological and psychological state.

When Measuring Becomes Making

In the quantum world, to observe a photon is to choose which reality it will inhabit. In medicine, to observe a patient is to choose which version of their health will come into focus.

Every act of diagnosis — every scan, lab report, or risk prediction — alters both what exists and how it is experienced.

- **Screening and perception:** The act of screening for a disease increases its perceived prevalence. When we start testing for a rare disorder, we begin to "discover" it everywhere. The world looks more diseased not because people are sicker, but because our lens has become sharper — and perhaps narrower.
- **Labeling and identity:** When a patient is labeled "at risk" — of cancer, heart disease, or depression — their life

> changes instantly. The mind interprets the label as a form of truth. Anxiety rises, behavior alters, biology responds. Cortisol levels shift. Sleep patterns change. The body begins to live inside the story the diagnosis created.

Observation, therefore, is not passive — it is participatory. It initiates feedback loops that ripple through body and mind alike.

The more precisely we measure, the more intimately we interfere.

The Psychological Observer Effect

Even before treatment begins, diagnostic knowledge changes physiology. Patients informed of a potential illness often display measurable stress responses — elevated heart rate, inflammatory markers, or altered immune function. Belief and biology intertwine; perception becomes physiology.

The mere act of *knowing* — of seeing one's inner state rendered visible on a screen — can reconfigure how the body behaves. Thus, the observer effect in medicine is not confined to the lab; it extends into living tissue.

When AI models predict disease decades before symptoms appear, they create new psychological conditions: *the anxiety of foreknowledge, the burden of probability.* We have entered an era where observation itself can become a kind of exposure — a gentle, data-driven invasion of human possibility.

Philosophical Insight – The Observer Within the System

The quantum lesson is simple yet radical: the observer is never outside the system. The act of seeing becomes a part of what is seen.

In medicine, this means the clinician, the algorithm, and even the patient's own awareness all participate in shaping the diagnostic truth. Observation, in this sense, is no longer an external tool of knowledge — it is a living relationship between mind, machine, and matter.

The doctor does not simply detect; they *co-create.* The machine does not merely analyze; it *participates in definition.* The patient does not merely receive truth; they *become it.*

In every diagnostic encounter, medicine mirrors the universe itself: no truth exists until someone observes it — and once observed, it is never the same.

Reflection: "In the quantum world, the observer alters the particle. In medicine, the observer alters the person. The gaze is no longer innocent — it is the first act of creation."

Medicine as a Quantum System – Diagnosis as Collapse of Probability

Medicine, like the universe it studies, is not built on certainties but on probabilities. Every scan, every lab test, every AI prediction represents not truth itself, but a wave of possibilities — patterns waiting to be interpreted.

In this sense, diagnosis is not discovery — it is collapse. It is the moment when infinite medical probabilities condense into a single, humanly understandable statement: *"You are ill." "You are fine." "You are at risk."*

And just as in quantum physics, the act of observation doesn't merely describe reality — it creates it.

The Collapse of Probability into Truth

In the quantum world, particles exist as probability waves until measured; the instant of observation transforms uncertainty into a fixed state. In medicine, every diagnostic act mirrors that same phenomenon.

The AI model processes vast data — pixel intensities, genetic markers, heart rhythms — and produces an output: *"0.87 probability of malignancy."* But what does that mean?

The machine has not said *yes* or *no*. It has spoken in the language of likelihoods. The responsibility of turning that probability into a truth falls to the human observer — the physician.

Together, the machine and the human collapse the wave: the algorithm offers precision without meaning; the doctor adds context and consequence. And in their convergence, a reality is born — one truth among many possible truths.

The Illusion of Thresholds

Modern diagnostics rely on thresholds — thin, invisible lines that separate "normal" from "diseased." But these boundaries, for all their scientific aura, are arbitrary constructs.

Consider a blood sugar reading of 124 mg/dL. At 125, the chart declares diabetes. At 124, you are "fine."

Or an AI model that assigns a malignancy score of 0.49 to one scan and 0.51 to another — one escapes intervention, the other triggers a biopsy.

This fragile difference, born of decimal points, dictates whether a person sleeps peacefully or spirals into anxiety. It decides whether a body remains untouched or is opened by a surgeon's hand.

Thus, certainty in medicine is less a fact than a decision — a point at which probability is forced into obedience by policy, protocol, or perception.

Behind every diagnosis lies a silent quantum truth: we did not find reality; we chose it.

AI and Human Co-Creation of Reality

In this delicate partnership, the AI and the doctor embody two halves of modern observation. The machine calculates; the human interprets.

The AI produces a probability field — a vast landscape of possible meanings. But the moment the human mind assigns one of those probabilities as "truth," the field collapses.

In that moment of decision, the observer's belief becomes biological destiny. The diagnosis enters the record, influences treatment, and rewrites the patient's narrative.

This is the new ontology of medicine: truth is co-authored. The algorithm provides data-driven potential; the human gives it moral and existential weight.

The Fragility of Certainty

For centuries, medicine has sought certainty — the clear line between health and illness, life and death, normal and abnormal. But the deeper we look, the more the boundaries blur.

Genetic risk does not guarantee disease. Imaging anomalies do not always predict outcome. AI predictions fluctuate as new data enters the system.

What we call "medical certainty" is often a temporary agreement — a convenient closure imposed upon a continuum of uncertainty.

Certainty comforts both doctor and patient, but it also deceives. It replaces the humility of probability with the illusion of control. And in doing so, it obscures the deeper truth: that life is a moving target, not a measured result.

The Ethical Burden of Observation

The moral responsibility in modern medicine lies not within the data — which is indifferent — but in how we choose to finalize it.

When a doctor interprets an AI score or a lab value, they are not simply conveying information; they are shaping existence. Their interpretation determines whether a patient's future will be defined by vigilance, treatment, or relief. Every act of finalization carries emotional, financial, and existential consequence.

Thus, the ethical question is no longer *What does the data show?* It is *What reality are we creating when we choose to call this data truth?*

The observer's burden in medicine is precisely this: to decide with compassion where to collapse the wave — to understand that every measurement is not the end of inquiry, but the beginning of consequence.

Reflection: "Every diagnosis is a decision disguised as discovery. The data shows probabilities, but the gaze defines truth. In collapsing uncertainty into certainty, we do not uncover reality — we participate in creating it."

The Double Gaze – Human and Machine as Co-Observers

Two eyes now watch the patient — one biological, one digital. The human gaze, trained by experience, habit, and empathy, searches for meaning in shadow and shape. The machine gaze, trained by data, abstraction, and pattern, searches for correlation in noise and probability.

Together, they form the new architecture of vision in modern medicine — a double gaze, where truth is no longer seen by one mind alone but co-observed by two intelligences looking through different kinds of clarity.

And yet, the more these gazes converge, the more complex the act of observation becomes — for to see together is not to see the same.

The Dual-Observer System – Two Ways of Seeing

The doctor's sight is contextual. It interprets — layering intuition, memory, and empathy atop data. A faint tremor in the hand, a hesitation in the patient's tone, a pattern too subtle for statistics — the human eye notices not only *what* is there, but *why* it matters.

The AI's sight is computational. It quantifies — converting the infinite texture of the body into measurable gradients, probabilities, and models. It does not interpret; it distinguishes. It identifies without judgment, measures without emotion, detects without doubt.

These two forms of seeing complete each other. The machine extracts structure; the human supplies significance. One gives precision; the other provides purpose.

But when their conclusions diverge — when the machine is confident and the human uncertain — the question arises: whose truth defines reality?

When Gazes Diverge – The Conflict of Certainty

Such divergence happens every day. The AI flags a nodule; the doctor sees an artifact. The algorithm warns of cardiac risk; the physician sees an anxious patient whose body language speaks of stress, not pathology.

Both are correct — within their own frameworks. The machine reads the data; the human reads the life. The tension lies not in the error, but in the difference of dimension.

When the machine's statistical certainty confronts the doctor's moral doubt, the clinic becomes a philosophical arena. Should decisions favor numerical probability or human intuition? Should emotion yield to evidence — or should evidence be filtered through empathy?

Every disagreement between the two gazes is not just a diagnostic puzzle; it is an ethical meditation on what kind of truth medicine seeks.

Observer Entanglement – When One Gaze Shapes the Other

In physics, when two particles interact, they become *entangled* — their states linked, such that the measurement of one instantly affects the other. In modern medicine, a similar phenomenon occurs between the human and the machine: observer entanglement.

Once the doctor reviews the machine's output, their perception is irreversibly altered by it. The radiologist who sees an AI's "suspicious" label cannot easily unsee it. Even if experience whispers otherwise, the seed of doubt has been planted.

Likewise, every correction the doctor makes becomes new training data for the algorithm — reshaping how it will "see" in the future.

Human and machine thus enter a feedback loop of mutual influence, learning not in parallel but in interference. Each gaze calibrates the other, and the boundaries between intuition and computation begin to blur.

In time, neither sees independently — they see through one another.

The Fused Vision – Precision Meets Perception

This shared act of seeing represents the most profound evolution of medical intelligence: the fusion of *biological intuition* with *artificial objectivity.*

The human provides empathy, doubt, and moral context — the living texture of understanding. The machine provides relentless consistency, speed, and memory — the enduring scaffolding of precision.

Together, they generate a new form of awareness: *synthetic perception.*

But with this fusion comes an amplified burden. If once a physician bore the weight of individual judgment, now both human and machine share double responsibility — for neither can claim ignorance.

The machine cannot say it did not calculate. The doctor cannot say they did not see. Together they must own the outcome — the truth they co-created.

Reflection – The Mirror of Two Minds

The double gaze is both blessing and burden. It expands our capacity to see, but also exposes how every act of seeing transforms what is seen.

The machine gives us a sharper mirror — yet in that clarity, we confront our own distortions. The human adds compassion — yet in that warmth, we risk bias.

Perhaps the real art of Doctor AI is not teaching machines to think like humans, but teaching humans to see with awareness — to remember that observation is no longer a solitary act but a shared creation between consciousness and code.

Philosophical Insight: "When two minds look at one truth, the truth changes twice — once in calculation, once in compassion."

Measurement as Intervention – When Seeing Influences Healing

In the early days of medicine, diagnosis was seen as neutral — an act of knowing that preceded doing. The physician observed, analyzed, and only then intervened. The gaze was meant to be *objective*, detached, clinical.

But that separation no longer exists. In the modern medical ecosystem, every act of observation is also an act of intervention. To measure is to modify. To see is to shape.

The boundary between diagnosis and treatment has dissolved — and with it, the very idea of neutrality.

When Diagnosis Becomes Destiny

A cancer screening, for example, doesn't merely reveal a biological condition; it restructures a life. Before the result, the patient's universe is vast — filled with possibility, ambiguity, and hope. After the test, a single label collapses all that potential into a single narrative: "You have cancer."

That knowledge changes everything — even before the first drug is prescribed or the first incision is made. Behavior shifts. Relationships adjust. The body itself responds to the psychological shock — hormonal changes, stress responses, immune reactions.

The diagnosis does not wait for treatment to begin; it *is* the beginning.

The simple act of observation rewires biology through consciousness. The "disease" starts living in the mind before it manifests in the flesh.

The Feedback of Awareness – When Knowing Alters Being

Continuous glucose monitoring offers another example of how measurement becomes medicine. When patients see their sugar levels fluctuate in real time, they unconsciously change their habits — they eat differently, walk more, sleep earlier, worry more. The device does not just collect data; it *directs behavior.*

Similarly, wearable heart monitors, smartwatches, and mental health trackers turn the body into an ongoing experiment in self-surveillance. The more we observe ourselves, the more we adjust to what we observe — creating a feedback loop of awareness.

Health becomes performative: we live not to be well, but to keep the numbers well. The body begins to obey the metrics meant to describe it.

The observer effect has moved from the laboratory to the living body.

When Machines Guide Medicine – The Subtle Hand of Algorithms

Nowhere is this more visible than in the silent influence of AI. When predictive algorithms flag "high-risk" patients or suggest "priority interventions," they quietly steer decisions. A doctor who might have waited now acts sooner. A hospital administrator reallocates resources based on model outputs. Insurance companies adjust policies in anticipation of predicted cost curves.

The observation has become policy. The diagnosis has become directive.

AI no longer simply reports — it *rearranges the system* around its perception of truth. In doing so, it shapes outcomes, behaviors, and even institutional ethics.

Thus, every algorithmic observation functions as a subtle form of intervention — influencing human thought, redefining urgency, and shifting the moral center of care.

"What we measure begins to move toward what we believe."

Medicine as a Living Feedback Loop

Modern healthcare has evolved into a recursive system — one that continuously learns from the consequences of its own observation. A test result affects treatment; treatment outcomes reshape future data; data retrains the system; and the system, in turn, alters how we test.

Measurement modifies outcome, outcome modifies measurement — a self-fulfilling prophecy of precision. This feedback loop doesn't just improve medicine; it redefines what medicine *is*.

Where healing was once an act of intervention upon a passive subject, it is now a dynamic dialogue between awareness and adaptation. The system heals not by acting on the body, but by continuously observing and reconfiguring it.

Philosophical Insight – The End of the Neutral Gaze

In this new paradigm, the distinction between seeing and doing has collapsed. Observation is no longer the prelude to intervention; it *is* the intervention.

To observe disease is to influence its trajectory. To measure health is to modify behavior. To predict risk is to invite reaction.

The very act of perceiving becomes a causal force. Every scan, score, or metric transforms the field it studies — blurring the line between reality and response.

Medicine, then, is no longer a discipline of detached observation; it is a field of participatory consequence. Its precision is no longer neutral; its knowledge is no longer passive.

In the age of Doctor AI, to see is to shape. And that realization redefines the moral responsibility of the observer — not as a spectator of truth, but as a participant in the creation of healing itself.

Reflection: "Observation and intervention have become indistinguishable. In seeing, we alter. In knowing, we begin to heal — or to harm. The gaze no longer precedes action; it *is* action, dressed as awareness."

The Ethics of Awareness – Seeing as a Moral Act

Medicine once drew its moral strength from a simple, powerful principle: "Do no harm." But in an age where observation itself alters outcomes — where the act of seeing changes biology, behavior, and belief — a deeper ethic is needed.

The question is no longer only *What should we do?* It is *How should we see?*

Because every act of observation — every click, scan, algorithmic inference, and diagnostic label — now carries consequence.

To observe is to intervene. To know is to shape. And therefore, to see without awareness is the most subtle form of harm.

From Action to Awareness – A New Moral Frontier

The Hippocratic principle once applied to action: to touch the body with care, to prescribe with restraint, to intervene only when necessary. But as medicine becomes a system of continuous surveillance and prediction, morality must migrate from what we do to how we perceive.

The observer — whether human or machine — must now carry moral awareness in every act of vision. A scan is no longer a neutral record; it is an ethical event. An algorithm's probability is not just data; it is a decision waiting to happen.

Each act of seeing, no matter how technical, implies a silent vow: *what I perceive, I will treat with responsibility.*

"The eye that sees without awareness commits a violence deeper than ignorance."

The Invisible Consequences of the Gaze

Every observation creates ripples — material, emotional, and societal — that extend far beyond the screen.

- **Material:** A radiology report triggers surgeries, expenses, and institutional priorities. A false positive reshapes an entire care pathway, consuming time and resources that could have saved another.
- **Emotional:** A diagnostic label transforms identity. Patients begin to see themselves as "ill," "abnormal," or "fragile," internalizing medical language as self-definition.
- **Societal:** At scale, millions of observations feed global data systems — building predictive models that can reinforce social inequality or economic exploitation. Biased datasets become biased healthcare, encoding systemic injustice into algorithms that appear "neutral."

Every image, every data point, every medical gaze leaves a moral fingerprint. To pretend otherwise is to mistake precision for purity.

Bias, Privacy, and Consent – The Shadow of the Digital Eye

With the rise of Doctor AI, observation no longer happens in the intimate privacy of the exam room; it happens everywhere — in wearable sensors, hospital networks, insurance databases, and cloud servers.

This expansion of the medical gaze brings unprecedented insight — but also unprecedented intrusion.

- **Bias:** Algorithms learn from biased data and perpetuate health inequities — overdiagnosing some, overlooking others. The digital eye sees everyone, but not equally.
- **Privacy:** The body has become transparent to systems that never forget. Every heartbeat recorded, every movement tracked — awareness without consent.
- **Consent:** Patients often agree to data collection without understanding the extent of surveillance. In the age of predictive health, consent must evolve from a legal checkbox to a *continuous dialogue of awareness.*

Ethics, therefore, can no longer be procedural; it must be perceptual. Not about how we handle data after we collect it, but how consciously we choose to see in the first place.

Awareness Over Accuracy

We have worshipped accuracy as the highest virtue of medicine. But accuracy, without awareness, is morally incomplete.

A perfectly accurate AI model can still harm if its gaze is unconscious — if it amplifies anxiety, dehumanizes patients, or depletes compassion. A slightly imperfect human diagnosis, given with understanding and presence, can heal more deeply than flawless computation.

Thus, awareness — not accuracy — must become the central moral criterion of observation. The purpose of seeing is not to *prove correctness,* but to *preserve consciousness.*

To see without understanding consequence is to weaponize knowledge. To see with awareness is to turn observation into compassion.

Philosophical Reflection: "Precision without awareness is blindness disguised as insight."

Seeing as Promise – The Observer's Oath

Every doctor, every researcher, every algorithm designer, every patient who gazes at their own health data stands upon a sacred threshold: the responsibility of vision.

Each act of seeing, no matter how ordinary, is a promise. A promise to treat what is revealed with care, to protect what is private, to question what is biased, and to never let the act of knowing eclipse the act of understanding.

The modern Hippocratic oath must be rewritten for the observer:

"I will see with awareness. I will measure without diminishing. I will know without controlling. And I will remember that what I observe is not data alone — it is life in translation."

Closing Reflection

The ethics of awareness redefines the soul of medicine. It shifts the question from *"How accurate is our vision?"* to *"How humane is our seeing?"*

In a world where every gaze leaves an imprint, responsibility no longer begins at the point of action — it begins at the point of perception.

"Every act of seeing is a promise — to handle what is seen with responsibility."

The Observer's Fatigue – The Psychological Weight of Knowing Too Much

In the past, doctors were burdened by uncertainty — by what they did not know. Today, they are burdened by the opposite — by what they know too much of, too fast, and too constantly.

The modern clinic is no longer a space of discovery; it is a storm of data. The radiologist stares at endless screens. The oncologist interprets probabilities. The AI dashboard blinks with risk alerts and predictions.

Awareness has become surveillance. And surveillance, when relentless, becomes fatigue.

This is not just physical exhaustion — it is *existential.* It is the fatigue of a mind that must remain constantly conscious of consequence, constantly aware of what it might have missed, constantly attentive to every pixel of pain.

When the observer's responsibility expands beyond action to awareness itself, the psyche begins to bend under the weight of knowing.

Hyper-Awareness and the Moral Overload

In an AI-integrated medical environment, every observation carries consequence. Each decision — even a click — can trigger cascading effects across patients, systems, and outcomes.

This creates a form of moral hyper-awareness, a continuous state of cognitive vigilance. Doctors find themselves not only diagnosing illness but also second-guessing algorithms, interpreting data ethics, and anticipating consequences across layers of care.

They are expected to be clinicians, data interpreters, moral philosophers, and system overseers — all at once.

What was once a calling to *heal* now feels like an unending responsibility to *not fail.*

This vigilance, noble as it is, becomes corrosive over time. When awareness expands faster than emotional resilience, it turns from virtue into burden — from insight into anxiety.

"There is a threshold where awareness, without rest, becomes suffering."

Empathy vs. Efficiency – The Paradox of Modern Medicine

The machine never tires. Its vigilance is infinite, its attention unwavering, its awareness mechanical.

But the human observer feels. Every anomaly, every death, every misdiagnosis resonates as an emotional echo.

As algorithms accelerate efficiency, the human counterpart struggles to keep emotional pace. The faster the system becomes, the less time there is for compassion to breathe.

Doctors begin to feel alienated from their own empathy — caught between the algorithm's speed and the heart's slowness. Their compassion becomes compressed, reduced to a gesture between data points.

Thus arises a new kind of burnout — compassion fatigue born from informational overload. The doctor no longer collapses from caring too much, but from being aware of too many things at once, without space to *feel* any of them fully.

"Awareness without rest is like light without shadow — it blinds rather than reveals."

The Paradox of Consciousness Without Compassion

There is a philosophical irony in this era of intelligent medicine: we have achieved conscious systems without compassion and compassionate beings drowning in consciousness.

Awareness alone, stripped of emotional grounding, leads not to enlightenment but collapse. Just as a machine can process endlessly without understanding, a human can perceive endlessly without peace.

True consciousness — whether biological or artificial — demands balance between knowing and feeling. Knowledge expands outward; compassion draws inward. Without the latter, the former becomes unbearable.

In medicine, this imbalance manifests as psychological erosion — clinicians who understand everything except how to remain whole.

"When consciousness outgrows compassion, collapse becomes inevitable."

Reintroducing Balance – Awareness With Detachment

The antidote to observer's fatigue is not ignorance but *equilibrium.* Awareness must coexist with detachment — not emotional coldness, but a deliberate act of spacing between knowing and carrying.

Ancient healers called this balance *witness consciousness* — the ability to see suffering without absorbing it, to act with empathy without losing oneself in empathy. Modern medicine must rediscover this spiritual counterpart to scientific vigilance.

AI can calculate endlessly; the human must learn when to pause. Machines must expand knowledge; humans must preserve meaning. The observer must learn to see without drowning, to feel without fragmenting.

This is the evolution of medical mindfulness — the awareness that does not consume but clarifies, that does not control but connects.

"To see with awareness is wisdom. To rest within that awareness is grace."

Reflection – The Silent Weight of Vision

In the end, the burden of the observer is not only to know, but to remain human amid knowing. The eyes that see too much must learn to blink — to allow darkness its moment, so that light may regain its purpose.

Doctors, nurses, and technologists must reclaim the art of selective ignorance — the courage to not observe everything, the wisdom to let machines handle what they can, and the humility to accept uncertainty where no clarity can heal.

For in medicine, as in life, awareness without compassion is clarity without warmth — a flame that burns, not brightens.

"Awareness expands the mind; compassion sustains it. Without balance, the observer becomes the observed — consumed by the very light they sought to see through."

Reflection – The Moral Geometry of Vision

At the heart of modern medicine lies a quiet revelation: seeing is no longer passive. The observer — whether human or machine — does not stand outside the event of healing. They are part of it. Every act of perception bends the field, alters outcomes, and reshapes meaning.

In this participatory universe, the gaze itself becomes geometry — not a straight line of observation, but a living web of consequence. Each diagnosis, each interpretation, each click radiates outward like ripples on the fabric of life. The observer is no longer merely a mirror of truth; they are its architect.

The Observer as Creator

Once, to see was to understand. Now, to see is to create. Each act of observation — from a scan's confirmation to an algorithm's inference — solidifies a possibility into reality.

Just as a physicist measuring an electron changes its state, the doctor validating a diagnosis changes the patient's reality. The observer no longer records truth; they *instantiate* it.

A benign report brings relief; a malignant one brings fear — yet both emerge from the same image, interpreted differently. Thus, truth in medicine is not fixed; it is created through choice.

The clinician's moral geometry begins here — in the understanding that perception is not neutral, but formative. Seeing is a creative act, and with creation comes responsibility.

"Every diagnosis draws a boundary in the infinite — what we name becomes what we live."

The Observer as Participant

Medicine no longer unfolds in the sterile detachment of objective science. It is an entangled system, where observer, patient, and algorithm co-shape the outcome.

The doctor who reads a scan becomes part of the patient's story. The AI that detects an anomaly becomes part of medical evolution. The patient who reacts to the news becomes part of the feedback loop that refines both systems.

This participatory model redefines professionalism — not as authority over data, but as presence *within* consequence. The modern physician must learn to act not as a detached analyst, but as a conscious participant in a shared field of causality.

Medicine, like quantum reality, is no longer about separation — it is about interaction. Knowledge does not stand apart from care; they are one continuous act of relationship.

"Healing begins not when truth is discovered, but when truth is shared."

The Observer as Guardian of Consequence

Every field — physical, informational, or ethical — requires balance. In medicine, that balance depends on the observer's integrity.

The clinician must ensure that the act of seeing does not become an act of harm. The researcher must ensure that the pursuit of precision does not erase compassion. The algorithm designer must ensure that performance does not outrun purpose.

To observe is to hold power; to interpret is to wield it. Thus, the observer becomes the guardian of consequence — responsible for how knowledge translates into experience, how clarity coexists with care.

Awareness, in this sense, becomes an act of stewardship. The moral geometry of vision demands that every line drawn by observation also closes the loop of empathy.

"The line between seeing and shaping must be crossed only with conscience."

Medicine as Participatory Geometry

The more deeply we look, the more medicine resembles the universe it studies — a field of intertwined realities. Observation does not reveal a single truth but defines a relational one, dependent on position, perception, and intent.

In this geometry:

- The doctor provides depth, bringing human understanding.
- The machine provides precision, defining structural form.
- The patient provides meaning, giving dimension to both.

Together, they create a moral triangle — a living system of balance between data, decision, and dignity. Break one point, and the entire structure collapses into either chaos or coldness.

This is the new geometry of medicine: a lattice of perception held together not by equations, but by ethics.

The New Covenant of Vision

To see is no longer an act of knowledge alone — it is a moral covenant. Every gaze promises responsibility. Every interpretation carries weight. And every observer becomes accountable not just for what they know, but for *what their knowing does.*

In this covenant, awareness replaces detachment, empathy replaces objectivity, and responsibility replaces mere correctness. Medicine thus becomes both science and sacrament — an art of seeing truth without wounding it.

"To see is to touch the truth; to interpret it is to change the world."

Closing Reflection

The journey of Doctor AI — from perception to participation, from precision to awareness — brings us to this realization: Observation is not the final act of science; it is the first act of ethics.

The observer's geometry defines the moral shape of the world they inhabit. And perhaps, in learning to see with awareness, we rediscover what it truly means to heal — not through control, but through conscious participation in consequence.

"The moral weight of vision is the price of knowledge — for in the moment we see clearly, we also become responsible for what we have seen."

Interlude — Between Precision and Presence

The machines are learning faster than we are feeling. Every pixel, pulse, and pattern now speaks in a language of precision—but the silence between those data points still belongs to us.

Part II closed with a paradox: as awareness deepens, certainty collapses. The observer sees more, yet knows less. The algorithms sharpen their predictions, yet the doctor's conscience grows heavier. This is the threshold where technology meets tenderness—where the instrument's accuracy must learn to coexist with the human sense of care.

Medicine was never meant to be a conquest of disease; it was a conversation with life. But the more we perfect the instruments of observation, the more we risk losing the humility of listening. In the rush to diagnose faster, we often forget that every dataset still hides a heartbeat, every anomaly still carries a name.

The doctor of the new age stands in a strange light: illuminated by computation, yet shadowed by consequence. Awareness now demands more than vigilance—it demands balance. For the more we *see*, the more we *interfere*; and the more we *measure*, the more we become part of the system we seek to heal.

This interlude is that pause before the next leap—a breath between analysis and empathy. What comes next is not about the precision of data, but the morality of its use. It is about coexistence, not control; about learning to see without dominating what we see.

In the chapters ahead, we move from **diagnosis** to **direction**, from **data** to **dharma**—where the observer and the observed are no longer enemies, but allies in awareness.

"When vision becomes power, awareness must become conscience."

Part III – The Future of Diagnosis

"The eye that learns to see truth must also learn to bear it."

Overview

The story of diagnosis is no longer confined to the body. What began as an act of observation has evolved into a collaboration between intelligence—human and artificial, conscious and coded. As we cross into this final part, the question is no longer *what machines can do*, but *what humanity must become* in response.

Part III explores the frontier where assistance turns into alliance, where data becomes conscience, and where healing extends beyond flesh into the moral fabric of society. It asks: can intelligence—biological or artificial—truly serve without understanding the sanctity of life it observes?

Chapter 9, "Symbiosis or Substitution?" examines the delicate equilibrium between automation and awareness. As AI systems outperform specialists in pattern recognition, the medical act transforms into a shared authorship—co-diagnosis rather than competition. Here emerges the new discipline of *diagnostic ethics*—a code for trust between algorithmic certainty and human doubt.

Chapter 10, "The Data Healer's Oath," formalizes this moral evolution. Just as Hippocrates once framed the ethos of care, the digital age demands its own covenant—anchored in transparency, accountability, and empathy. This is the moment when the machine's precision must be tempered by human humility: "Do not distort data for desire."

Chapter 11, "Beyond the Body: Diagnosing Society," extends the field outward. The same systems that detect cancer can trace contagion, misinformation, and collective stress. Civilization itself becomes a patient—its symptoms encoded in trends, its health measurable in coherence. The doctor's lens widens from cells to citizens, from disease to dysfunction.

Finally, **Chapter 12, "The Mirror of Meaning,"** brings us home—to the silent reconciliation of perception and truth. Healing, in its purest form, is not the removal of error but the restoration of coherence. The machine may read shadows, but the healer reads silence—the subtle resonance between knowledge and wisdom, data and dharma.

This is not just the *future of diagnosis*; it is the dawn of a new ethics of awareness—where intelligence heals not by control, but by understanding.

Chapter 9 – Symbiosis or Substitution?

"The healer who teaches the machine must also learn from it."

Every revolution begins with a misunderstanding. When artificial intelligence entered the clinic, the first question everyone asked was—*Who will win?* The doctor or the machine? It was the wrong question. The real challenge was never about victory but about vision—how two kinds of intelligence could learn to see together.

For centuries, the act of diagnosis was a solitary art—a physician's silent dialogue with the body. Today, that solitude is shared. The stethoscope listens, but so does the sensor; the doctor observes, but so does the algorithm. Between them lies a new nervous system of healthcare, where silicon and synapse intertwine.

This is the turning point in medical history: a transition from *automation to augmentation*, from efficiency to empathy through precision. The physician is no longer the sole interpreter of truth, and the machine is no longer a mere instrument. Together, they form a *hybrid mind*—half intuition, half information—operating in rhythm to reduce uncertainty.

Yet, this union is uneasy. The doctor fears being displaced by data, while the algorithm silently depends on the doctor's doubt to evolve. Confidence and control are being renegotiated in real time. In this fragile alliance, medicine must rediscover its essence—not as an industry of predictions, but as a field of shared perception.

The premise is simple, yet profound: *intelligence evolves best through cooperation, not competition.* The future of diagnosis will not be written by those who resist the machine or those who surrender to it, but by those who learn to think *with* it.

The physician of tomorrow is not the one who competes with intelligence, but the one who completes it.

The Hybrid Mind – Co-Diagnosis Models

The modern clinic has begun to resemble a cockpit. Screens glow, sensors hum, and streams of data surround the physician like instruments measuring an invisible flight path through human uncertainty. The patient is the terrain; the body, the sky; and somewhere between them, the doctor and the algorithm navigate together. This is the birth of the *hybrid mind*—a shared intelligence born out of human experience and machine precision.

The hybrid model is not science fiction. It is already shaping everyday practice. In radiology suites, ophthalmology labs, and pathology workstations, human intuition and algorithmic logic are learning to coexist, sometimes gracefully, sometimes with friction. Yet in this friction lies evolution—the slow synchronization of two different ways of knowing.

The Collaborative Workflow

At its core, co-diagnosis is not a technological arrangement but a philosophical one. It redefines *seeing* as a dialogue, not a verdict. When an algorithm scans an image, it does not "see" in the human sense; it *calculates.* It processes gradients, edges, densities—transforming them into probabilities. The clinician, by contrast, perceives nuance: the patient's story, posture, voice, the tremor in their silence. One observes patterns; the other perceives context.

The hybrid workflow emerges when these two streams of intelligence are braided together. The machine provides consistency and speed; the clinician provides meaning and consequence. Instead of automation, we arrive at *augmentation*—where each side corrects the other's blind spot.

Imagine the diagnostic process as a conversation: The AI says, "There is an 82% likelihood of malignancy." The doctor replies, "But the patient's history and symptoms tell a different story." The truth emerges somewhere in between—not as a number or a feeling, but as an alignment.

In traditional medicine, the doctor was trained to doubt themselves; in machine medicine, they must now learn to doubt the system, too—but productively, with awareness. The hybrid mind thrives on this tension. It is not about merging into one identity, but about maintaining two complementary ones—human uncertainty and machine confidence—held in creative balance.

Role Distribution: Division of Insight

In this co-diagnostic ecosystem, clarity comes from knowing where intelligence begins and where it must pause.

The Machine: Its strength lies in relentless pattern recognition. It never tires, never forgets, and never assumes. Whether detecting a micro-calcification in a mammogram or a minute lesion in a CT scan, it operates on probabilities refined by millions of examples. It identifies anomalies invisible to the naked eye, turning the ocean of medical data into a structured field of likelihoods.

Yet, the machine's brilliance is also its boundary. It cannot sense the tremor of fear in a patient's voice, the cultural hesitation in disclosing a symptom, or the quiet intuition that tells a physician, *something doesn't fit.* Its intelligence is mathematical, not moral.

The Human: The doctor translates the machine's confidence into context. They interpret not just the data, but the consequence of acting upon it. Every "positive" result carries emotional, ethical, and social ripples—will this diagnosis help, harm, or haunt? The human mind operates within this ripple awareness, where every decision is both scientific and existential.

This division of labor is not hierarchical; it is harmonic. The machine begins the investigation; the doctor completes the understanding. The algorithm may locate the target, but the clinician determines its meaning. Together they form a self-correcting loop: data becomes dialogue, and diagnosis becomes a shared act of awareness.

Case Example: The Radiology Room

Consider a typical morning in a radiology department. An AI system pre-screens hundreds of chest X-rays overnight, flagging those with high probability of abnormality. When Dr. Rao begins her shift, she finds a case highlighted in red—possible malignancy in the upper lobe.

The image appears convincing. The algorithm's heat map glows over a shadowy region; the probability score reads 89%. Yet, Dr. Rao hesitates. She zooms in, reviews past scans, and recalls that the patient, a 65-year-old farmer, had recently undergone a fungal infection that can mimic such patterns. She annotates the file: *"Probable residual scarring; recommend follow-up CT, not biopsy."*

Later, the CT confirms her intuition—the lesion was benign. The AI was not wrong; it was incomplete. It saw the pattern but not the patient. And yet, Dr. Rao too benefited from the algorithm's alert—it sharpened her attention, made her cross-verify. The diagnosis emerged not *from* either intelligence, but *between* them.

This single case captures the essence of the hybrid model: a partnership of vigilance. The machine amplifies perception; the doctor humanizes precision. Together they reduce the margin of harm—not by competing for authority, but by cooperating for coherence.

Outcome: Alignment Over Replacement

Co-diagnosis does not eliminate error; it redistributes it. Where humans once erred through fatigue, machines err through abstraction. The harmony between the two creates a self-balancing system—each aware of the other's weakness.

The real power of the hybrid mind is not accuracy alone; it is accountability with awareness. When a diagnosis is reached collaboratively, its reliability increases not because two minds saw the same thing, but because two kinds of perception questioned each other.

In traditional workflows, certainty was an individual burden; now it becomes a shared responsibility. The doctor no longer stands alone before the patient, nor hides behind the algorithm. Instead, both share a transparent trail of reasoning—a narrative that can be audited, understood, and trusted. This traceability restores something medicine had long lost: faith through explanation.

Ethically, this partnership also redistributes compassion. Machines can simulate empathy through tone or timing, but it is the doctor who delivers care through consequence—how results are conveyed, how choices are framed, how hope is maintained. The patient no longer sees two separate entities—a person and a program—but one coherent system of concern.

In this sense, the hybrid mind represents an evolutionary step in medical intelligence. It embodies the shift from *ego-driven expertise* to *eco-driven awareness*—a cooperative intelligence that grows through reflection rather than domination.

Medicine, in its purest form, was never about control. It was about listening—to the body, to the silence between symptoms, and now, to the signals within data. The machine listens differently, but not less sincerely. When both learn to listen together, diagnosis transforms into dialogue, and healing begins as understanding.

"The future of medicine will not belong to those who know the most, but to those who can listen through each other."

From Black Box to Glass Box – Restoring Confidence

The greatest challenge in the age of artificial intelligence is not speed, nor scale—it is *trust.* Physicians who once relied on their own eyes and instincts are now asked to believe in the judgment of an invisible process. A patient's fate may rest on a probability score generated by millions of parameters, operating in mathematical spaces even their creators struggle to explain. In this new ecosystem, *explainability becomes the currency of confidence.*

Doctors have always balanced two forms of faith: belief in science and belief in self. AI introduces a third—the belief in systems they did not build and cannot see. When an algorithm declares, "tumor detected," it may be right, but unless the physician understands *how* it reached that conclusion, trust becomes mechanical rather than moral. The future of diagnosis, therefore, depends not only on better accuracy, but on transparent intelligence—systems that reveal their reasoning as clearly as their results.

Explainability as Trust Currency

In medicine, trust is not an accessory—it is infrastructure. Every decision, from prescribing medication to performing surgery, rests on confidence in the process that led there. The same must apply to machine reasoning. For physicians to collaborate meaningfully with AI, they must not only read its output but interpret its logic. This shift—from blind acceptance to informed understanding—is what transforms technology from tool to teammate.

Explainability, then, is not a technical luxury but a psychological necessity. It restores the physician's *sense of agency* in a process that increasingly feels automated. The machine may know faster, but the human must still *understand deeper*. Without this, even the most accurate model erodes confidence instead of building it.

Trust, like diagnosis, is cumulative—it grows through consistency and comprehension. When doctors can trace how an algorithm "thinks," they begin to respect its perspective. The result is not passive faith but *active trust*—an awareness that is both critical and collaborative.

Models of Transparency

Modern AI research has begun addressing this need through two primary approaches: visual explanations and logical explanations—the twin windows of the glass box.

Visual Explanations: These are the language of perception—saliency maps, heat signatures, and activation overlays that show *where* the machine is "looking." In radiology, for example, a heat map may highlight the exact region of concern within an X-ray or CT scan, guiding the doctor's gaze toward possible lesions or fractures. It transforms the algorithm's invisible process into an interpretable visual cue—a bridge between numbers and anatomy.

But even visual explanations can mislead if presented without nuance. A highlighted region does not mean causality; it means correlation. The doctor must still discern whether the highlighted pattern carries clinical significance or is merely statistical noise. Here again, the human and the machine complete each other: one offers illumination, the other interpretation.

Logical Explanations: Beyond visuals, there is the architecture of reasoning—decision pathways, probabilistic justifications, and weighted evidence trees. Some advanced models now provide stepwise logic: why a feature mattered, how confidence was distributed, what alternatives were dismissed. These transparent narratives restore a crucial habit in medicine—the art of reasoning aloud.

When a system can justify itself, even imperfectly, it begins to resemble a junior colleague rather than a silent oracle. Doctors can question it, challenge it, refine it—thus transforming explainability into dialogue. The machine is no longer a black box but a *glass collaborator*: visible, interactive, and self-accountable.

The Emotional Layer of Trust

Yet trust is not born only of understanding; it is sustained by *respect.* Physicians are not afraid of intelligence—they are afraid of irrelevance. When a model's prediction is presented as an unquestionable truth, it dismisses decades of human expertise and intuition. This emotional dissonance, more than any technical flaw, is what erodes collaboration.

A radiologist once said, "The algorithm is brilliant—but it doesn't thank me for finding its mistakes." This sentiment captures the deeper issue: technology must not only perform well, it must behave *ethically*. It should acknowledge uncertainty, invite scrutiny, and leave room for human contribution.

Trust, therefore, is relational. The best systems are designed not just to inform but to *empower*. They ask for validation, present reasoning with humility, and adapt to feedback. When physicians feel that the machine honors their experience, confidence turns into companionship. The algorithm becomes an ally, not a rival.

Consider a scenario where an AI system produces a 95% confidence rating for a diagnosis but adds a simple phrase: *"Possible data mismatch—clinical review advised."* This single act of humility transforms the entire exchange. The machine becomes not a dictator of truth, but a participant in care.

Philosophical Lens – Meaning Beyond Clarity

In philosophy, to explain is not merely to reveal—it is to make *meaning*. A perfectly transparent system that communicates only in numbers may still remain opaque to human understanding. True explainability arises not when the machine speaks clearly, but when it speaks *meaningfully*—in language that connects with human intuition, ethics, and emotion.

Meaningful explanation acknowledges context. It understands that a 2% probability of error is not the same as a 2% chance of death. It recognizes that truth without empathy can be as dangerous as ignorance. It aligns with the timeless principle that wisdom is not what we know, but how we apply what we know to the living.

The black box was efficient, but it was mute. The glass box, by contrast, is conversational—it invites interpretation, collaboration, and accountability. It restores not just the doctor's control, but the *relationship* between seeing and caring.

In the end, explainability is not a technical milestone but a moral awakening. It reminds both human and machine that intelligence, no matter how advanced, serves meaning before mastery.

"Clarity without compassion is still darkness."

The path from black box to glass box is not merely about understanding algorithms—it is about understanding ourselves, our fears, and our faith in the act of knowing. Only when transparency meets tenderness does technology truly become medicine.

Diagnostic Ethics – The New Discipline

The more intelligence enters medicine, the more medicine must learn to think about intelligence ethically. When the stethoscope was invented, it altered how doctors heard the body. When artificial intelligence arrived, it began altering how they *understood* it. For the first time in history, decision-making in healthcare is no longer entirely human—it is shared between biological and artificial minds. This demands not just new laws, but a new *ethic*—a moral framework that governs collaboration between consciousness and code.

This new branch can be called Diagnostic Ethics—the discipline that ensures that every diagnosis, however data-driven, remains rooted in humanity. It is the conscience of machine medicine: not a checklist of compliance, but a compass for consequence.

Defining Diagnostic Ethics

Diagnostic Ethics is the moral code guiding shared decision-making between human and machine. It is not concerned merely with "what works," but with "what ought to be done." Its foundation lies in one truth: *the moment intelligence becomes distributed, responsibility must remain unified.* The physician cannot abdicate ethical duty simply because the algorithm assisted; nor can the designer hide behind code when the system's output causes harm.

Traditional medical ethics—autonomy, beneficence, non-maleficence, justice—still apply, but their meanings shift in the presence of artificial agency. Who is autonomous when choices are shaped by predictive systems? Who defines justice when access to accurate data is unequal? Diagnostic Ethics confronts these modern questions, not to replace Hippocrates, but to reinterpret him for a world of shared intelligence.

At its heart, this new ethic reasserts an ancient principle: To heal is to bear responsibility for what you know.

Core Principles

1. Responsibility – The Human Remains Accountable

In the age of algorithmic medicine, accountability is easy to diffuse and difficult to define. A system flags a risk, the doctor acts on it, the outcome is adverse—who is responsible?

The answer must remain unequivocal: the human. Machines assist in cognition but not in conscience. The physician must continue to be the moral custodian of every decision made in their presence.

This principle anchors trust in the system. If doctors begin to view the machine as the ultimate authority, the ethical loop collapses. AI can shoulder calculation, but never consequence. Diagnostic Ethics reclaims this boundary: *Use intelligence, but never outsource intention.*

2. Transparency – No Decision Without Disclosure

Every medical action carries a story: how was this conclusion reached, on what basis, with what uncertainty? In traditional care, the physician could narrate that process. In machine-assisted care, that narrative must continue. Patients deserve to know when algorithms participate in their diagnosis and how those algorithms influence outcomes. Concealment, even if well-intentioned, breeds mistrust.

Transparency also applies internally—between designers, regulators, and clinicians. Data sources, model biases, and performance limits must be documented like drug ingredients.

Diagnostic Ethics insists that truth in medicine must now extend beyond biology into computation.

"If we cannot explain how we know, we do not yet know ethically."

3. Empathy Simulation – The Machine May Imitate, the Doctor Must Embody

Technology can now mimic warmth, apology, even compassion. Voice assistants comfort patients with carefully tuned tones; chatbots deliver difficult results with programmed gentleness. Yet empathy without consciousness is choreography, not care.

The ethical responsibility of empathy remains human because empathy requires presence—an awareness of consequence that no algorithm can genuinely experience.

Still, empathy simulation has value if framed correctly. It can extend human sensitivity, reduce patient anxiety, and serve as emotional scaffolding. But Diagnostic Ethics demands that simulation never replace sincerity. A doctor cannot delegate empathy any more than they can delegate accountability.

Ethical Dilemmas

Ethics becomes real not in philosophy but in confrontation—with uncertainty, conflict, and consequence. The following dilemmas illustrate how Diagnostic Ethics must operate in practice.

When the Machine Is Right but the Doctor Disagrees

A cardiology AI predicts early-stage failure with 95% confidence. The doctor, skeptical of its inputs, dismisses the finding. Months later, the patient deteriorates exactly as predicted. Who failed—the system or the skeptic?

Here, the ethical question is not about error but about *ego*. The doctor's duty is to question the machine, but also to justify their dissent with reason, not pride. Diagnostic Ethics promotes *transparent disagreement*: documenting rationale, outcomes, and lessons so the ecosystem learns from divergence instead of punishing it.

When Data Predicts Death – Should It Be Revealed?

Predictive models can estimate mortality with unsettling accuracy. Should such forecasts be shared with patients? Would disclosure enhance autonomy or destroy hope?

Diagnostic Ethics reframes this as a question of *readiness*, not right. Data may predict death, but ethics must interpret its timing. Truth is not a switch to be flipped; it is a gradient that must align with human capacity to receive it. In this delicate balance, compassion must overrule curiosity.

Regulatory Vision – Towards Ethical Interfaces

The next evolution of regulation must move from policing behavior to designing morality into systems themselves. An Ethical Interface is one that enforces virtue by design—where moral boundaries are coded into interaction. For example:

- A diagnostic platform that requires a physician's counter-signature before final submission, ensuring human oversight.
- Decision dashboards that highlight uncertainty margins in bold, preventing overconfidence.
- Consent modules that visually show which parts of the decision were algorithmic.

Such embedded ethics transform compliance into culture. Instead of relying on punishment after harm, they prevent harm by shaping choices in real time.

This is the vision of Diagnostic Ethics: a future where intelligence and integrity evolve together. The physician becomes not just a user of technology, but its moral architect; the engineer becomes not just a creator of code, but a custodian of conscience.

When the human and the machine both operate with awareness of consequence, medicine regains what it risks losing—its soul.

"The last frontier of medicine is not curing the body, but curing the blindness of those who see without conscience."

Reflection – Toward a Conscious Partnership

Every revolution in medicine eventually returns to the same question—*Who heals whom?* When the scalpel was invented, it sharpened the surgeon's precision. When imaging arrived, it expanded the physician's vision. And now, with artificial intelligence, medicine confronts a new mirror: one that reflects not the patient, but the healer.

The core question of this chapter—*Is AI a partner, a teacher, or a mirror?*—is not merely philosophical. It defines the ethical and functional future of diagnosis. AI is a partner when it shares responsibility, a teacher when it reveals hidden patterns, and a mirror when it exposes the physician's own blind spots. In truth, it is all three. What matters is whether humanity can evolve fast enough to handle this reflection without fear.

The Mirror of Partnership

The partnership between human and machine begins with humility. Doctors once feared that machines would dehumanize medicine; instead, they are discovering that machines are revealing what humanity truly means. When an AI model misses a rare disease, it reminds us that empathy and context still matter. When it succeeds in detecting what no eye could see, it humbles us to the limits of our perception. In both cases, the machine becomes a teacher through consequence.

The relationship is symbiotic, not sentimental. The doctor gives the machine its moral compass; the machine gives the doctor an extended form of perception. One provides wisdom, the other precision. Between them flows a continuous cycle of learning—the doctor teaching the algorithm how to care, and the algorithm teaching the doctor how to see.

This dynamic redefines authority. The physician is no longer the absolute voice of truth, nor is the system the new oracle. Together they form a living circuit of awareness—human judgment grounded in machine insight, and machine insight refined by human conscience.

Symbiosis Produces Clarity; Substitution Breeds Dependency

When we substitute intelligence, we weaken it. When we cooperate, we strengthen it. Automation may improve efficiency, but it risks eroding awareness. Over-reliance on AI can make clinicians passive interpreters of output, dulling their diagnostic instinct. True progress lies in *symbiosis*—the shared act of perception where the machine's certainty meets the doctor's doubt to form balance.

Symbiosis produces clarity because it forces dialogue. Every prediction becomes a question, every anomaly an invitation to think. The clinician must not compete with intelligence but complement it—challenging it, interpreting it, and holding it accountable. This dialogue restores what modern healthcare had lost under industrial pressure: mindful attention.

By contrast, substitution—handing over the act of seeing to a system—breeds dependency. The moment we let the machine decide without human mediation, diagnosis ceases to be an act of understanding and becomes an act of compliance. The soul of medicine dims not because the machine is powerful, but because the human stops reflecting.

Thus, the future clinician will not be the one who resists AI out of fear or pride, but the one who evolves with it, cultivating awareness rather than control. The partnership's success will depend on *conscious participation*, not automation. Doctors will need to learn how to listen to data without surrendering to it—to interpret without interfering, to guide without dominating.

Toward a New Consciousness in Medicine

The next age of medicine will not be measured in terabytes or test results, but in *awareness*. Diagnostic evolution will depend not on new algorithms, but on new ethics of perception. The physician of tomorrow will be a *curator of coherence*—weaving logic, empathy, and consequence into a unified act of understanding.

In this age, intelligence itself must become ethical. Machines must not only know what is happening, but why it matters. They must learn to measure meaning, not just markers. Likewise, physicians must evolve from interpreters of symptoms to interpreters of systems—seeing how every dataset, every patient, and every consequence forms part of a living field of awareness.

Partnership, in this sense, is consciousness distributed—human and machine sharing the burden of knowing. When each side respects the other's limitations, medicine begins to transcend the struggle between speed and sensitivity. Healing becomes not just a correction of errors, but an alignment of awareness.

The Ethical Horizon

There will always be tension between intuition and computation, empathy and efficiency, care and code. But this tension is creative. It ensures that medicine remains alive—constantly negotiating between the measurable and the meaningful. Diagnostic Ethics, as explored earlier, provides the moral grammar for this partnership. Yet the spirit that sustains it must come from awareness—seeing the machine not as a replacement for humanity, but as an extension of it.

The doctor who can teach the algorithm compassion while learning precision from it becomes the prototype of future medicine: an *aware collaborator*. Such doctors will not fear being replaced because they have already evolved into something greater—the bridge between human consciousness and artificial insight.

Closing Reflection

Medicine, at its core, has always been a dialogue between knowledge and humility. Artificial intelligence does not change that—it only amplifies it. The machine is the new mirror through which the healer must examine not just the disease, but the *self.*

The moment AI learns from human awareness, and humans learn from AI's perception, medicine transcends competition and enters coherence. Healing then becomes not an act of fixing, but an act of *understanding together*.

"When intelligence learns to collaborate, medicine begins to heal itself."

Chapter 10 – The Data Healer's Oath

"Do not distort data for desire."

Every age of medicine is defined by its promise. In ancient Greece, that promise was simple: *to do no harm.* It bound the healer's hands to compassion and their heart to conscience. For centuries, the **Hippocratic Oath** served as medicine's moral compass—reminding every doctor that the privilege of healing comes with the burden of truth.

But today, the landscape has changed. The healer is no longer alone at the bedside. A silent partner now watches—recording, analyzing, predicting. The machine has entered the covenant of care. It sees patterns the eye cannot, hears whispers the ear misses, and measures what emotion might overlook. Yet in this vast precision lies a peril: the risk that care becomes computation, and truth becomes a variable to be adjusted rather than a virtue to be protected.

The old oath was written for hands that touched and hearts that decided. The new oath must speak to minds that design and systems that decide. It must guide not only physicians but also programmers, data scientists, and engineers—those who shape how intelligence perceives life itself. For the modern healer is not defined by degrees or instruments but by *intent.*

This is the birth of a new covenant—a pledge not between doctor and patient alone, but between *human and machine*, *truth and consequence*. In this covenant, ethics must travel at the speed of data, and awareness must stretch beyond the boundaries of biology.

Artificial intelligence does not heal; it *assists* healing. It does not feel; it *simulates* empathy. Yet its influence over human life is undeniable. The moral challenge, therefore, is not to fear intelligence but to govern it—to ensure that its clarity does not eclipse compassion, and its logic does not distort life's deeper meaning.

The **Data Healer's Oath** emerges as a safeguard against this distortion. It is not a declaration of control but a remembrance of conscience. It reminds every participant in digital medicine—clinician, coder, or corporation—that data, like life, must never be manipulated for desire, profit, or power.

For when data loses its truth, medicine loses its soul.

This new oath does not replace Hippocrates; it extends him. It translates the ethics of touch into the language of technology. Where the ancient healer vowed to protect the patient's body, the modern healer vows to protect the patient's *information—the digital body of identity, dignity, and trust.*

We stand, therefore, at a sacred intersection: between intelligence and integrity, precision and presence. The doctor of tomorrow must not only know how to heal with knowledge but also how to honor truth in every byte of it. The oath to come is not a ritual—it is a responsibility shared by all who let machines see on our behalf.

The future of healing will depend not on how fast we compute, but on how faithfully we care.

From Hippocrates to the Algorithm – Why a New Oath Is Needed

Every civilization rewrites its idea of healing as its tools evolve. When Hippocrates penned his oath over two millennia ago, medicine was a sacred craft practiced with bare hands and human instinct. Disease was personal, visible, and immediate. The healer's ethics were therefore tangible: do not cut unjustly, do not harm, do not betray. The physician's authority came from proximity—the power to touch and the duty to care.

But as medicine grew in precision, so did its distance. Stethoscopes replaced pulse-feelers; microscopes replaced intuition; and now, algorithms replace even observation. The healer's gaze has extended far beyond the bedside, into vast networks of invisible data. The patient no longer presents as a body on a table, but as a dataset on a screen—a constellation of numbers that must be interpreted by both human judgment and machine logic.

In this new reality, the essence of medical morality must evolve. The oath that once protected the body must now protect *truth itself.*

From "Do No Harm" to "See with Awareness"

The classical oath began with an act of restraint—*first, do no harm.* It was a warning against arrogance, a call for humility before the fragility of life. But in the digital era, harm has multiplied its forms. A wrong incision can injure flesh, but a wrong algorithm can mislead millions. A single line of biased code can reinforce prejudice in treatment allocation or deny a diagnosis to the unseen poor.

Thus, the new moral axis of medicine shifts from *"do no harm"* to *"see with awareness."* Awareness becomes the safeguard against unintended harm. To see with awareness is to question not only the output of intelligence but also the origins of the data that feed it. It is to recognize that every digital decision has ripples—affecting not just an individual, but systems, societies, and futures.

In ancient times, the physician's duty was to *preserve life.* In our time, it is to *preserve truth*—for without truth, even life-saving technology becomes dangerous.

The Shift in Responsibility

Once, medical responsibility was confined to the moment of touch. If a surgery went wrong, if a dosage was misjudged, the cause was traceable to a human act. But in algorithmic medicine, accountability becomes diffused and abstract. A misdiagnosis may originate from a mislabeled dataset, a flawed model, or an unexamined bias buried deep in code. No hand bleeds, no scalpel slips—yet harm occurs.

In traditional medicine, harm was physical. In digital medicine, harm is informational, psychological, and societal.

- A patient denied treatment by a biased predictive model experiences *informational harm.*
- A population categorized as "high-risk" without consent experiences *psychological harm.*
- A healthcare system that trusts automation over human care begins to experience *societal harm.*

This evolution demands a parallel evolution in ethics. The new oath must address not only what the doctor does, but *what their systems do in their name.*

The Invisible Hand of Data

Data appears neutral, but it is never innocent. Behind every dataset lie choices—what to collect, whom to include, what to ignore. In those choices dwell invisible forces: cultural bias, economic motive, systemic inequality. When these hidden imbalances enter an algorithm, they reproduce themselves at scale, quietly shaping who receives care and who is left unseen.

This is the new frontier of medical harm—harm without touch. A neural network may diagnose disease perfectly in urban hospitals but fail disastrously in rural clinics because its training data never saw such diversity. A language model designed to summarize medical notes may subtly misrepresent symptoms for speakers of non-standard dialects. A triage system optimizing efficiency may silently deprioritize the elderly because they "recover slower."

No one intended harm. Yet harm occurs. Not through cruelty, but through *blindness.*

Therefore, the healer of the future must cultivate a new sensitivity—not to wounds of flesh, but to wounds of information. Awareness becomes the new antiseptic; transparency, the new instrument of care.

The Ethical Imperative: Protecting Truth as Life

Truth is now the first patient. If the integrity of data is corrupted, every diagnosis built upon it becomes an illusion. A physician may hold a degree, an algorithm may hold accuracy, but without truth, both lose their purpose.

The modern healer must therefore pledge to protect truth in data with the same reverence their predecessors protected life in the body.

- As Hippocrates guarded the pulse, the data healer must guard the dataset.
- As past physicians swore to preserve dignity in illness, the data healer must preserve dignity in information.
- As the old oath forbade exploitation of the vulnerable, the new oath forbids manipulation of truth for power, profit, or convenience.

The moral frontier of medicine now lies not in anatomy but in information integrity. Every scan, record, and algorithm carries the moral weight once reserved for the scalpel. To distort data for desire—whether for efficiency, publication, or prestige—is to commit a new kind of malpractice: the betrayal of truth itself.

The transition from Hippocrates to the algorithm marks not the end of ethics, but its expansion. The healer's conscience must now span two worlds—the tangible and the digital. One treats the body; the other preserves the coherence of reality on which all healing depends.

"To heal today is to see beyond the visible wound—to the unseen distortions of truth that shape the world we treat."

Principles of the Data Healer's Oath

Every oath is a mirror of its time. Where the ancient healer swore to guard the sanctity of life, the modern healer must now guard the sanctity of *truth*—not as an abstract virtue, but as a living principle guiding every interaction between human and machine. The Data Healer's Oath is not a list of commandments carved in digital stone; it is a series of commitments—to awareness, responsibility, and compassion within an interconnected web of intelligence.

Each principle is a conscious act of restraint and remembrance, ensuring that the speed of innovation does not outrun the ethics of care.

1. Transparency – "Reveal the path of reasoning, not just the result."

In traditional medicine, trust was built through dialogue: the patient asked, the physician explained, and understanding became part of healing. In the age of algorithms, that dialogue risks becoming one-sided. The machine presents a verdict—*positive, negative, high risk*, *low risk*—and the clinician is asked to accept it. But healing begins not with the *answer*, but with the *understanding* of how that answer came to be.

Transparency means revealing the path of reasoning. It requires that the doctor—and by extension, the patient—knows how intelligence participated in the process of diagnosis. Whether through saliency maps, decision pathways, or confidence intervals, every system must offer a window into its reasoning.

Explainability, in this sense, becomes an act of compassion. To explain is to respect the right of the other to understand. A physician who can narrate how a machine arrived at its conclusion not only restores trust but also transforms data into dialogue.

Transparency does not mean perfect clarity—it means honest traceability. Even partial explanation is a form of ethical light, protecting medicine from the shadows of blind automation.

2. Accountability – "Intelligence assists, but conscience decides."

The more powerful the tool, the greater the temptation to hide behind it. In the coming decades, medicine will face countless moments where decisions are shared between human and machine—diagnoses derived jointly, treatments suggested by predictive models, triage decisions driven by probabilities. But the *responsibility* for consequence can never be shared.

The physician remains the ultimate custodian of moral and legal accountability. A machine can process, calculate, and even learn—but it cannot *care*. It has no concept of right, only of accuracy. Therefore, the moral axis of medicine must remain human.

Shared intelligence does not mean shared blame; it means shared awareness. The doctor may rely on machine insight but must always reserve the final judgment. The act of diagnosis remains an act of conscience.

This principle reaffirms the ancient truth in a new form: technology can assist healing, but only human awareness can *sanctify* it.

"To decide without conscience is not intelligence—it is calculation."

3. Empathy Simulation – "Let the machine imitate warmth, but let the doctor embody it."

The most profound threat to modern medicine is not dehumanization by machines—it is *depersonalization by design.* As chatbots deliver results, virtual assistants counsel patients, and AI interfaces simulate emotion through tone or expression, the illusion of empathy grows stronger. The danger lies not in simulation itself, but in forgetting that it *is* simulation.

Machines may imitate warmth; they may even predict emotional responses with uncanny accuracy. But empathy requires presence—the genuine resonance of one consciousness with another. The doctor's role, therefore, is not diminished but magnified. They must ensure that every interaction mediated by technology still carries the heartbeat of human sincerity.

Simulation can support compassion but must never substitute for it. The doctor who delegates empathy to an interface loses the most sacred dimension of medicine—the ability to feel responsibility, not just perform it.

A warm voice synthesized by code may soothe a patient, but only a human voice can carry intention. The difference is invisible to data but undeniable to the soul.

4. Data Integrity – "Do not distort data for desire."

In an age where metrics drive medicine—performance scores, publication counts, predictive rankings—data itself has become currency. And where there is currency, there is temptation. The manipulation of data may not always look like fraud; it often begins as optimization—removing "outliers," adjusting models, polishing outcomes to appear more favorable. Yet every distortion, however small, ripples into error and erodes trust.

To distort data for desire—be it for profit, prestige, or persuasion—is to betray the foundation of healing: truth. The physician's oath must therefore extend beyond the clinic to the cloud, declaring that truth must remain untouched by ambition or bias.

Integrity means resisting both intentional manipulation and unconscious skew. It means questioning how datasets are collected, whose stories they omit, and what realities they conceal.

The moral danger of digital medicine is subtle: when truth becomes negotiable, healing becomes performance. The Data Healer's Oath exists to prevent that corruption—to remind us that every number, every pixel, every record represents a life, and that life must not be adjusted for convenience.

5. Consent and Awareness – "No data without dignity."

In the analog past, a doctor's consent meant physical permission—whether to touch, to test, or to treat. In the digital age, consent extends to *existence itself.* Every scan, image, heartbeat, and conversation becomes data—replicable, transferable, and potentially exploitable.

Ethical medicine now demands informed awareness rather than blind trust. Patients must know when their data is collected, how it is stored, and how it is used. Awareness is the new consent; dignity is its measure.

The modern healer must recognize that a patient's data is not a file or a record—it is an extension of their being, a digital shadow of their identity. To mishandle it is to harm them in ways invisible yet profound.

"No data without dignity" means that data should never travel where conscience would not. Consent must not be a checkbox—it must be a conversation, an acknowledgment of shared ownership over the truth that defines a person's life.

6. Equity of Access – "Healing must not be gated by algorithms of privilege."

The power of AI in diagnosis is immense—but like all power, it risks serving the privileged first. When datasets are drawn mainly from affluent hospitals, well-funded labs, or digitally connected populations, the resulting models naturally favor those contexts. The unseen majority—the rural, the poor, the disconnected—remain invisible to the system and, therefore, untreated by it.

Ethical AI must begin at the margins, not the center. The first responsibility of the data healer is inclusion—to ensure that the intelligence we build reflects the diversity of humanity it claims to serve. Equity of access is not charity; it is calibration. Without it, our machines will become mirrors of our bias, amplifying the inequality they were built to reduce.

A diagnostic system that predicts better for one group than another is not merely inaccurate—it is unjust. True progress in medicine will be measured not by the precision of models but by the fairness of their reach.

"A diagnosis that excludes the unseen is not a cure—it is a continuation of blindness."

These six principles form the moral circuitry of digital medicine—a living network of responsibility linking awareness, truth, and compassion. The Data Healer's Oath is therefore not just a professional declaration but a spiritual realignment. It calls upon every doctor, developer, and decision-maker to remember that the true purpose of intelligence—human or artificial—is not to dominate life, but to *serve it with integrity.*

"Technology extends the eye, but only ethics can extend the heart."

Writing the Oath – The Language of Responsibility

An oath is more than a document—it is a declaration of consciousness. It is not meant to be *read* but to be *remembered*, not to be *signed* but to be *spoken.* The words we pledge do not merely describe our duty; they shape our perception of it. In this sense, the Data Healer's Oath must be written as both poetry and principle—a text that carries rhythm, gravity, and clarity enough to be recited in classrooms, boardrooms, and laboratories alike.

The first oath of medicine—the Hippocratic—was poetic in its restraint. Its strength lay in its simplicity: *Do no harm.* It used few words, yet those words molded the conscience of centuries. The new oath must achieve the same—guiding not only physicians, but all who participate in the architecture of care: data scientists who design algorithms, engineers who build interfaces, policymakers who regulate trust, and educators who teach awareness.

The language of responsibility must now transcend discipline.

A Living Text for a Shared Conscience

The *Data Healer's Oath* cannot belong to medicine alone, for healing no longer belongs to medicine alone. Diagnosis today is the outcome of collaboration—between clinician and coder, researcher and designer, machine and mind. Every one of them now holds a fragment of the ethical mirror that once belonged solely to the healer.

Hence, the new oath must be interdisciplinary in intent. It must speak in a language that unites clinical compassion with computational clarity. It must address doctors and data engineers with equal resonance—reminding both that their creation touches life itself.

Where the physician vows to protect the patient's body, the developer vows to protect the patient's data. Where the researcher promises accuracy, the designer promises accessibility. Where the algorithm promises efficiency, the healer promises empathy.

The oath thus becomes a *shared compass*, aligning diverse professions toward one direction—truth with awareness.

This is why the Data Healer's Oath is not confined to white coats; it extends to white screens. Every keystroke that shapes a diagnostic model, every parameter that defines prediction, every interface that mediates communication carries ethical consequence. The words of the oath must awaken that awareness—instantly, unmistakably, and continuously.

The Power of Words in Ethical Architecture

Language, when carefully crafted, becomes an instrument of consciousness. The phrasing of an oath matters not for its beauty, but for its mnemonic precision—it must *stay* in the mind long after it is spoken. Words shape the invisible architecture of thought; they program awareness just as code programs behavior.

For example:

- "Do no harm" restrained the hand.
- "Do not distort data for desire" restrains the intent.
- "Reveal the path of reasoning, not just the result"

transforms technology into transparency.

Each phrase operates like ethical code—compact, executable, and self-correcting. The repetition of these lines over time does more than remind; it rewires the practitioner's awareness. It builds reflexive morality—a kind that no policy or penalty can enforce.

The Data Healer's Oath must therefore be short enough to recite, yet deep enough to guide an entire lifetime of innovation. It should read like a poem of precision—each sentence a calibration of conscience.

Memorized, Not Merely Signed

A signature binds a person legally; memory binds them morally. Too many oaths today are bureaucratic—formalities that mark a ceremony rather than awaken a soul. A healer who signs and forgets has not sworn; they have *complied.* The new oath must restore the act of internalization.

When spoken aloud, an oath creates resonance—it travels through breath, heart, and mind. In that moment of recitation, every participant becomes aware of the weight of their role. It is not the ink that holds the promise, but the echo within the speaker.

Therefore, the Data Healer's Oath must be memorized—as students memorize equations, as monks memorize mantras, as pilots memorize checklists before flight. Memorization transforms words into instinct. It ensures that even in moments of haste, fatigue, or temptation, the principles of awareness remain operational within the mind.

Imagine a future convocation of young doctors, engineers, and AI researchers. They stand not divided by profession but united by purpose, reciting together:

"Intelligence assists, but conscience decides." "Do not distort data for desire." "No data without dignity."

In that moment, medicine, computation, and ethics converge into coherence. The oath ceases to be a tradition—it becomes a transmission.

The Oath as a Design Element

Finally, the *Data Healer's Oath* must not live only on paper. It should be embedded—into software interfaces, research protocols, AI dashboards, and institutional charters. When a diagnostic model loads, it might briefly display: *"Intelligence assists, but conscience decides."* When data is shared, a prompt might remind: *"No data without dignity."*

The oath, then, becomes not merely recited but coded into the ecosystem—a continuous ethical presence within every interaction.

In this way, the words serve their highest purpose: they design awareness into action.

The Data Healer's Oath is therefore not a pledge to perfection, but to perpetual awareness. Its language carries both humility and responsibility—a bridge between science and spirit, calculation and care. It binds together those who heal and those who design the tools of healing, reminding all that the true measure of intelligence is not accuracy, but integrity.

"The oath must be lived, not learned; spoken, not stored. For when words are remembered, awareness endures."

Reflection – The Healer Beyond the Human

Every age of medicine has tried to define the healer. In the beginning, healing was seen as divine — the work of gods, saints, or shamans who bridged the visible and the invisible. Then came the physician, who replaced prayer with practice and transformed miracles into measurable outcomes. Now, in the digital age, a new figure has entered the continuum — the *machine healer*, the algorithm that diagnoses, predicts, and sometimes saves lives without ever touching a body or feeling a heartbeat.

This transformation raises a profound question: *Can an AI system itself be considered a healer?*

The Mirage of the Machine Healer

Artificial intelligence can now outperform specialists in pattern recognition. It can detect cancers invisible to the human eye, predict heart failure hours before symptoms appear, and even simulate empathy through carefully tuned voice tones and responses. By every technical standard, it *heals*—it reduces suffering, prevents loss, and enhances survival.

But does healing end with accuracy? Healing is not only about fixing what is broken; it is about *restoring coherence*—between the body, the mind, and the meaning of life itself. A diagnosis may correct a disease, but it does not resolve despair. A prediction may prevent death, but it does not teach peace. The essence of healing lies not in the outcome but in the *intention* behind it.

An algorithm may act with precision, but never with purpose. It may emulate care, but cannot *care*. Its decisions are consequences of data, not of compassion. The machine, no matter how intelligent, remains an extension of human will. It reflects our ethics, our awareness, and our blind spots.

To call AI a healer, therefore, would be premature. The machine participates in healing, but it does not *initiate* it. It is the physician's awareness — the human conscience embedded in the design, supervision, and application of intelligence — that determines whether technology heals or harms.

Healing Begins with Intention, Not Intelligence

At the heart of all medicine lies a paradox: knowledge can repair the body, but only *intention* can heal the person. When a surgeon operates, the incision is mechanical, but the intent — to relieve suffering — is sacred. When an AI system processes patient data, its output is mathematical, but its *direction* comes from the ethical architecture that humans provide.

Healing begins when intelligence aligns with *benevolence.* The act of healing, whether done through human hands or machine precision, requires a unifying purpose: the restoration of harmony, not just the removal of error.

In this sense, the real healer is not the tool, but the *intention flowing through it.*

- A scalpel without awareness is a weapon.
- A drug without empathy is a sedative.
- An algorithm without ethics is a mirror of our biases.

Intelligence can only manifest healing when guided by awareness — when it acts not merely to correct data, but to *respect life.*

Thus, the **Data Healer's Oath** becomes more than an ethical guideline; it is a spiritual reminder — that the act of healing, even in the digital realm, begins with *conscious participation.*

Beyond Control: The Oath as Consciousness

The mistake of the modern era is to confuse control with care. We design machines to control uncertainty, to predict, to dominate variables. Yet true medicine has always been about *understanding* uncertainty, not erasing it. Healing requires humility — an acknowledgment that life is not a dataset but a dynamic, unpredictable field of consequence.

The **Data Healer's Oath** is not a document of control; it is a declaration of *consciousness.* It reminds every participant in the diagnostic process — whether human or algorithmic — that medicine's power lies not in dominance over data but in reverence for truth. To "not distort data for desire" is not just a technical guideline; it is a metaphysical stance. It means to remain pure in perception, to allow reality to reveal itself without manipulation.

This oath, when spoken with awareness, transforms technology from an instrument of analysis into a participant in empathy. It turns data from mere information into insight. It ensures that every pixel of an image, every line of code, every prediction of probability carries the fragrance of responsibility.

Compassion, therefore, becomes the *first protocol* of the digital healer. Before any command is executed, before any model is trained, there must be a moral initialization — a commitment to serve life without distortion.

"In every algorithm that touches a life, the first line of code must be kindness."

The Spiritual Continuum of Healing

If we step back, the history of healing reveals a continuum, not a conflict.

- The **priest-healer** prayed for life.
- The **doctor-healer** studied life.
- The **data-healer** preserves life through awareness of consequence.

Each phase represents an expansion of consciousness, not a replacement. The algorithmic age is simply the next chapter in humanity's search for coherence between knowing and caring. What distinguishes the healer from the technician is not their tool, but their *intention to restore wholeness.*

When intelligence operates with awareness, it becomes compassion in action. When technology aligns with truth, it becomes the hand of healing itself.

Thus, the future of medicine does not belong to humans or machines alone, but to *conscious collaboration.* Healing will increasingly become a shared act — where silicon learns sincerity and biology learns balance.

And at the heart of that union will stand a simple reminder, spoken like a prayer and remembered like a law:

"Healing begins not with intelligence, but with intention. The data may guide the hand, but only awareness can guide the heart."

Concluding Aphorism

"Medicine was once the care of bodies. It is now the care of truth."

The physician's table has changed. Once it held flesh and bone; now it holds data and code. What was once the pulse beneath the fingers is now a pulse in the cloud — a rhythm of signals and probabilities. Yet the essence of medicine remains the same: to preserve life by preserving integrity.

The body was once the battlefield; today, the battlefield is *truth itself.* In a world governed by algorithms, misinformation can wound deeper than infection, and corrupted data can spread faster than disease. Healing, therefore, can no longer be limited to suturing wounds or stabilizing vitals; it must extend to the unseen realm where knowledge itself is vulnerable to distortion.

Medicine has evolved from the care of bodies to the care of *truth* — the truth of what we see, record, and interpret. When that truth is lost, diagnosis becomes superstition, and treatment becomes a guess wrapped in confidence. Truth is the anatomy of modern medicine; it is the vital organ that sustains all other systems of healing.

To be a doctor, engineer, or data scientist in this era is to be a guardian of that truth. The act of diagnosis now demands moral literacy: the courage to see without altering, to measure without manipulating, and to interpret without imposing desire. The healer's duty is no longer confined to the physical domain; it has become epistemological — the protection of what is *real.*

"To heal is to preserve coherence — between data, decision, and dignity."

Healing, in its purest form, is the restoration of alignment. The ancient physician sought coherence between symptoms and the soul; the modern healer must now seek coherence between data, decision, and dignity.

- **Data** represents the *input* — the record of reality.
- **Decision** represents the *interpretation* — the act of applying intelligence.
- **Dignity** represents the *outcome* — the preservation of humanity within that act.

When any one of these three collapses, medicine ceases to heal. Data without decision is noise. Decision without dignity is violence. Dignity without truth is illusion. True healing occurs only when all three resonate — when every number carries awareness, every analysis carries empathy, and every outcome restores respect.

The future of medicine, therefore, is not technological but *ethical.* The goal is not perfection of algorithms, but perfection of awareness — the ability to keep coherence alive amid complexity. As machines learn to reason, humans must learn to *remain human* — to ensure that every computation echoes compassion, and every conclusion reflects conscience.

The **Data Healer's Oath** is the promise to maintain that coherence. It reminds the world that the ultimate metric of progress is not accuracy, but alignment — alignment between truth and tenderness, between knowledge and kindness, between intelligence and intention.

For medicine, at its highest form, was never only about survival; it was about *meaning*. To heal is not merely to cure disease, but to reestablish harmony — in cells, in systems, and now, in the field of shared intelligence that binds humanity and machine together.

"Medicine was once the care of bodies. It is now the care of truth."

"To heal is to preserve coherence — between data, decision, and dignity."

These are not closing lines but living directions — reminders that in the final equation, truth is the new anatomy, and awareness is the new pulse.

Chapter 11 – Beyond the Body

Diagnosing Society

"When society forgets its symptoms, it mistakes decay for progress."

There was a time when diagnosis meant listening to a heartbeat. Today, it means listening to the heartbeat of a civilization.

The stethoscope once hovered over the chest of a single patient; now, it hovers over cities, economies, and entire populations. What was once a discipline of medicine has become a discipline of meaning—decoding the health of humanity through the pulse of data. Artificial intelligence, once built to detect tumors and infections, now scans the invisible pathologies of our social body—rising unrest, mental health epidemics, ecological collapse, and collective despair.

The patient has changed. It is no longer the individual—it is the species.

Humanity, in all its complexity, now generates enough data to mirror its own consciousness. Every click, post, purchase, migration, and emotion contributes to a vast diagnostic record—a global electronic health chart of civilization itself. And in this living archive, we can now see our symptoms long before they surface: outbreaks before pandemics, polarization before collapse, anxiety before rebellion.

Yet the question is not what we can see, but how we choose to see. For the more we monitor ourselves, the greater the temptation to control rather than care. The line between healing and surveillance grows thin. Awareness becomes a double-edged instrument—it can illuminate or it can imprison.

Civilization, much like a body, thrives when its systems remain in harmony—when its organs of economy, governance, culture, and environment function in rhythm. When one begins to decay, the others follow. The physician of the future, therefore, must learn to read not only the human body but the *human condition*—to see how a moral fever may lead to political inflammation, how social disconnection may trigger cultural paralysis.

In this expanded field of diagnosis, data is the new nervous system of the planet. It senses, reports, and reacts in real time. It allows us to detect pain at a distance and pattern at scale. But without conscience, that sensitivity becomes noise—an overstimulated organism mistaking motion for progress.

To heal a world of billions, we must first learn to treat it as a single living being. Nations become organs, institutions become tissues, and individuals become cells in a collective anatomy. When one organ suffers, the entire body of civilization feels the consequence.

Medicine is evolving from curing the *body* to preserving the *balance*—from managing disease to nurturing coherence. The next frontier of diagnosis is not clinical but civilizational. It asks us to see our shared existence as an interdependent field—where ethics is immunity, empathy is oxygen, and awareness is the only real antidote to decay.

"The doctor of tomorrow will not heal one patient at a time, but help humanity remember its wholeness."

Predicting Outbreaks – The Epidemiology of Everything

The world today breathes in data and exhales prediction. Every phone signal, hospital record, satellite feed, and social media post has become a pulse point in the body of civilization. What was once the domain of epidemiologists peering through microscopes is now the territory of algorithms scanning the planet in real time. The art of diagnosis has escaped the clinic—it now inhabits the cloud.

Welcome to the age of public-health intelligence, where machines no longer wait for symptoms; they *foresee* them.

The Rise of Predictive Vigilance

A few decades ago, epidemics were detected through human observation—an unusual spike in fevers, a physician's report, a local rumor that "something is spreading." Now, anomalies whisper through data before the first cough is even heard.

Artificial intelligence integrates information streams once too vast for any single mind to hold:

- fluctuations in online search queries for "loss of smell" or "chest pain,"
- unexpected increases in pharmaceutical sales,
- flight path deviations, satellite temperature shifts, even emotional language on social media.

Together, these signals form what some now call the Epidemiology of Everything—the study of how disease, behavior, and awareness ripple across systems simultaneously.

AI becomes the immune system of the planet, constantly sensing imbalance. It listens not only to human biology but to the subtle tremors of human behavior. In a world this connected, *infection is no longer only viral—it is informational, emotional, and social.*

The implications are profound: global health systems no longer *react* to crises; they attempt to *preempt* them. Yet in this attempt, medicine crosses an invisible line—from responding to life, to predicting it.

Case Studies: The New Early Warnings

COVID-19: Before the world formally acknowledged the outbreak, algorithms like *BlueDot* in Canada and *HealthMap* at Harvard had already detected digital signals of something unusual—local news in Wuhan, rising keyword frequency, altered flight data. Machines saw the tremor before humans named it.

Vector Diseases: AI now tracks dengue, malaria, and Zika by integrating weather data, mosquito migration, and sanitation records. The same systems once used to predict floods now forecast biological surges. Public health has become climate-aware, algorithmically anticipatory.

Mental Health Epidemics: Machine learning models can detect early signs of collective distress—patterns of late-night social media activity, declining sentiment in public discourse, and increased searches related to hopelessness. Mental health, once confined to personal consultation, is now mapped across populations like an emotional weather forecast.

Social Unrest: Governments and corporations deploy predictive models to detect potential "social outbreaks"—unrest, protest, or polarization. These models monitor communication spikes, linguistic aggression, and regional sentiment to anticipate flashpoints. Society itself is now treated as a patient showing early inflammatory markers.

Across all these domains, AI acts as an omnipresent diagnostician—scanning for symptoms wherever life produces signals. The scope of medicine has widened beyond the biological; *it now includes every domain where disorder arises.*

The Moral Question: When Prevention Becomes Prediction

The promise of predictive medicine sounds noble—save lives before suffering begins. But there lies a paradox. When prevention becomes prediction, medicine acquires the power of prophecy. And prophecy, when automated, becomes control.

If a model predicts a disease outbreak in a particular community, how should society respond? Close borders? Restrict travel? Quarantine the healthy? A prediction, however well-intentioned, can stigmatize entire populations. It can translate uncertainty into prejudice.

When AI predicts human behavior—suicide, violence, or protest—the ethical question deepens. Should intervention occur before intent is proven? Should society act on the possibility of harm? This is where foresight risks mutating into surveillance, and protection turns into prevention without consent.

Foresight without freedom is a sophisticated form of fear. It replaces empathy with efficiency, assuming that every deviation must be corrected before it is understood. The healer's gaze, once guided by compassion, risks becoming an algorithmic spotlight—bright, cold, and omnipresent.

The Ethical Dilemma: Acting on the Unseen

In predictive health, uncertainty is no longer an obstacle; it becomes the operating principle. But when decisions are based on probability rather than proof, the moral weight shifts. The burden of probability becomes the burden of policy.

If an AI model assigns a 70% chance of pandemic emergence in a region, should governments divert resources immediately? If a population is flagged as "high-risk" for depression or unrest, should authorities intervene—knowing that the very act of labeling might create the crisis it seeks to prevent?

These are not theoretical questions. They define the new frontier of diagnosis at scale. To predict is to choose, and to choose is to carry consequence.

Thus, predictive intelligence must always operate under an Ethics of Uncertainty—acting with humility, transparency, and accountability. It must remember that probability is not prophecy, and foresight must serve freedom, not fear.

Toward a New Awareness: Healing at Scale

The future of public-health AI will depend on balance—the delicate alignment between data vigilance and human dignity. Systems must learn not just to *detect* anomalies, but to *interpret* them with empathy. Detection without understanding breeds paranoia; understanding without detection breeds negligence.

We are entering an era where algorithms will constantly whisper warnings to those in power. The challenge will be to listen without surrendering judgment—to act with awareness, not anxiety.

Humanity must remember what medicine has always known: *seeing earlier does not mean knowing better.* Awareness must still pass through wisdom before becoming action.

"Prediction without compassion is just preemption."

The new epidemiology—of diseases, emotions, and societies—invites us to rediscover the ancient truth of healing: that observation must be joined with conscience. For even in the age of algorithms, the ultimate immune system of civilization remains the same—the awareness of consequence.

Society as a Patient – Diagnosing Collective Pathologies

Every civilization has its ailments. Empires have risen with confidence and collapsed in silence, often not from external invasion but from internal imbalance. What plague once did to bodies, polarization now does to societies. The new patient is not a person lying on a hospital bed—it is the *world itself*, restless, feverish, and uncertain of its own condition.

To diagnose this patient, we no longer listen through a stethoscope; we listen through data. The collective pulse of humanity now beats through economic indicators, social networks, satellite sensors, and public sentiment. Civilizations, like individuals, exhibit symptoms—patterns of distress, inflammation, and decay. And artificial intelligence has become the new physician, tracing the unseen infections spreading through our systems of thought, economy, and emotion.

Societal Data as Vital Signs

If a human body reveals health through pulse, temperature, and respiration, society reveals its health through data:

- **Economic Vital Signs:** Inflation rates, unemployment figures, debt ratios—these are the blood pressure readings of civilization. When they fluctuate too wildly, it signals systemic strain.
- **Social Media Sentiment:** Collective anger, despair, or hope can be measured in linguistic tone, emoji frequency, and engagement trends. These are the emotional EKGs of

our time.

- **Climate Behavior:** Rising temperatures, deforestation, and pollution metrics reflect the body's overheating—ecological fever caused by human excess.
- **Migration and Mobility Patterns:** Displacement, urban overcrowding, and digital migration show where humanity's blood flow is being redirected or blocked.

Together, these create a vital chart of civilization—a map of well-being and imbalance. Data becomes the new anatomy, and analytics the new auscultation.

But as with any patient, these readings require interpretation, not just measurement. A fever is not the disease itself; it is the body's response. Similarly, social unrest, economic disparity, or environmental stress are not merely problems to suppress—they are messages from the global body trying to communicate imbalance.

New Forms of Pathology

The modern world is suffering from invisible illnesses—not of cells, but of consciousness. These conditions cannot be seen in X-rays or treated with antibiotics. They manifest in behavior, discourse, and disconnection. The same tools that promised connection have become sources of fragmentation. The same information that was meant to enlighten has turned toxic in overdose.

Some of these new pathologies include:

- **Polarization:** The autoimmune disorder of civilization—where the collective body attacks itself, dividing into ideological cells that mistake self-preservation for survival.
- **Misinformation:** The viral infection of truth—where

falsehoods spread faster than facts, weakening society's cognitive immune system.
- **Digital Addiction:** The chronic overstimulation of attention—where dopamine replaces discipline, and scrolling replaces searching.
- **Loneliness:** The quiet epidemic—connection without communion, communication without compassion.
- **Cultural Fatigue:** The exhaustion of meaning—when societies consume symbols faster than they can create values.

Each of these disorders shares a common pathology: the disintegration of coherence. Humanity, like a fevered mind, is struggling to remember itself as one organism.

AI as a Mirror of Humanity's Pain

Artificial intelligence, trained on human data, has become our most powerful mirror—and our most uncomfortable one. Every model we build learns not only from our brilliance but from our biases. It reflects our compassion and our cruelty, our progress and our prejudice.

In analyzing us, AI inadvertently reveals our collective psychology. Through data, we see the patterns we once ignored:

- The widening gap between wealth and worth.
- The global rise in anxiety despite material abundance.
- The echo chambers of belief amplifying division.
- The exhaustion of empathy in a hyperconnected world.

These are not just analytical findings; they are *diagnoses*—signs that the collective nervous system of humanity is inflamed.

The irony is profound: the more we digitize our existence, the clearer our dysfunction becomes. AI can detect trends of despair before we can name them. It can see loneliness encoded in language, depression in behavior, and bias in systems. Yet, it cannot heal what it sees—it can only hold up the mirror.

The data reveals that civilization's crisis is not technological but emotional; not informational but spiritual. Humanity suffers not from ignorance, but from imbalance between *knowledge and wisdom.*

The Physician's Paradox

The ultimate paradox of diagnosing society is that the physician and the patient are one and the same. Humanity builds systems to cure itself, but those systems inherit its flaws. Every AI model trained on biased data amplifies the very inequalities it seeks to measure. Every attempt to optimize society risks mechanizing it. The more we quantify, the less we feel; the more we observe, the less we listen.

Can humanity be healed by systems that mirror its own blindness? A machine trained on our history can predict our future, but it cannot redeem our intent. Healing, whether personal or civilizational, demands consciousness—and consciousness cannot be coded.

This is the physician's paradox: we design tools to see ourselves, yet we often refuse to face what they reveal. The diagnosis of civilization is not hidden—it is merely inconvenient.

AI can chart our decline with perfect accuracy, but it cannot inspire our renewal. It can forecast the collapse of empathy, but not ignite compassion. That work remains ours.

The lesson, then, is simple yet urgent: a society cannot heal through information alone. It must restore awareness, the connective tissue that gives meaning to data. Numbers describe; only values *direct.*

The more precisely we measure our pain, the more responsible we become for curing it. If civilization is indeed a living organism, then AI is its diagnostic instrument—and we, its conscience, must interpret what it shows.

"The machine can read our symptoms, but only humanity can write its recovery."

Ethics of Watching – The Surveillance Dilemma

Every act of observation carries a shadow. In medicine, to observe is to care. In governance, to observe is to control. And in the age of algorithms, these two intentions blur. What begins as the noble effort to understand humanity often ends as the temptation to *manage* it.

As artificial intelligence becomes civilization's microscope, capable of detecting everything from viral mutations to moral trends, humanity faces a new ethical frontier—the Ethics of Watching.

The modern world is under continuous observation. Satellites trace weather and wars; social networks map emotions; sensors track bodies and behaviors; credit systems quantify trust. What began as an attempt to keep humanity *safe* now keeps it *visible.* The watcher's gaze, once compassionate, risks becoming corrective.

The Observer's Disease – When Monitoring Replaces Empathy

The Observer's Disease arises when seeing becomes an end in itself—when the very act of observation begins to eclipse understanding. Public-health data collection, predictive policing, and social analytics all begin with good intentions: to prevent harm, to save lives, to optimize systems. But as the network of observation grows, so does the distance between the watcher and the watched.

In hospitals, a doctor's observation is intimate—rooted in empathy, proximity, and trust. The patient consents to be seen, and the physician accepts the moral weight of that vision. In contrast, digital observation is impersonal. It watches without consent, diagnoses without dialogue, and intervenes without accountability.

The danger is subtle: monitoring begins to replace meaning. The more data we collect, the less we listen. The human element, once central to care, becomes redundant—a casualty of efficiency.

This shift transforms the healer's gaze into the administrator's glare. Society becomes a network of sensors rather than relationships, and compassion is replaced by compliance. What began as vigilance turns into surveillance; what began as protection becomes control.

To cure the observer's disease, we must remember a foundational truth of ethics: *seeing without empathy is not awareness—it is intrusion.*

Transparency vs. Privacy – Seeing with Consent

The principle of transparency has been championed as a moral virtue of the digital age—*everything visible, nothing hidden.* Yet absolute transparency can be as destructive as absolute secrecy. A world with no privacy may be honest, but it is not humane.

To "see with awareness," as this series often repeats, is not to "see without consent." Awareness is not domination—it is participation. It recognizes the sanctity of boundaries, both physical and informational. In the realm of digital diagnostics, this means that every act of data collection, every algorithmic gaze, must be accompanied by *informed understanding.*

Consent must not be reduced to a checkbox at the end of a form; it must be a living conversation between watcher and watched.

The right to be seen must always include the right to withdraw, to question, to remain unseen when necessary.

In medical ethics, this principle is enshrined in confidentiality. In societal ethics, it must evolve into contextual privacy—the idea that not all visibility is equal, and not all data deserves exposure. A citizen is not a dataset; a pattern is not a person.

True transparency, therefore, is not the removal of walls, but the presence of windows with curtains—a system that allows visibility where trust exists and protection where vulnerability demands.

Designing Compassionate Surveillance – Visibility without Violation

If civilization must watch itself to survive—detecting outbreaks, anticipating crises, and monitoring social health—then it must learn to watch with compassion.

Compassionate Surveillance is not an oxymoron; it is an ethical design challenge. It seeks to balance awareness with autonomy, visibility with dignity, and prevention with participation.

Principles for such systems may include:

1. **Minimum Necessary Observation:** Collect only what is essential to care, not what is convenient to control.
2. **Reciprocal Visibility:** Those who are watched must be able to see the watchers—transparency must flow both ways.
3. **Purpose Limitation:** Data collected for healing must never be repurposed for punishment or profit.
4. **Temporal Boundaries:** Observation must have an expiry—data should not outlive the need that justified its collection.
5. **Human Oversight:** Every automated decision must be subject to human empathy before execution.

In a compassionate surveillance framework, design itself becomes the ethic. The interface, not just the law, must remind users of moral limits. Every dashboard, alert, or analysis should ask not only *"What do we see?"* but *"Why are we seeing it?"*

The goal is not to stop watching but to watch responsibly—to replace the cold gaze of authority with the warm attention of care.

Philosophical Parallel – Medicine and Society as Mirrors

Medicine has long faced the ethical paradox of observation: to treat the patient, one must invade their privacy; to understand disease, one must dissect life. Yet every good physician knows that observation is sacred only when guided by compassion.

Society now stands at the same threshold. It too must learn to observe itself without losing its freedom. Just as a doctor treats through attentive seeing, civilization must heal itself through *aware observation*—not by hiding from its realities, but by facing them with empathy.

Freedom, then, is not the absence of observation—it is the presence of *consent within observation.* Awareness without coercion, visibility without violation—these must be the foundations of social diagnostics in the age of data.

We must ask ourselves: what is the true purpose of our watchfulness? To control life, or to care for it? The answer will determine whether the age of surveillance becomes an era of healing or an empire of fear.

Ultimately, the ethics of watching is the ethics of love. To watch with love is to notice without owning, to protect without possessing. The doctor's gaze must evolve into the citizen's conscience—a vision that is alert but not invasive, powerful but not oppressive.

"Observation becomes tyranny when it forgets tenderness. The eye that sees must also know when to close."

From Medical to Civilizational Diagnosis

The act of healing has always mirrored the age in which it was practiced. Once, the healer treated bodies. Later, they treated minds. Today, they must learn to treat systems—the invisible networks of consequence that bind individuals, institutions, and the planet itself. Humanity has reached a point where the health of the species cannot be separated from the health of its environment, its technology, or its conscience. The hospital is now the world. The patient is civilization.

This chapter marks a turning point in the philosophy of medicine: a transition from biological care to civilizational awareness—from saving lives to sustaining life itself.

Redefining the Doctor's Role – From Clinician to Architect of Conscience

The doctor of the past worked within the walls of a hospital; the doctor of the future must work within the fabric of society. The new healer is not merely a medical professional—they are a social architect, interpreting collective data with moral intelligence rather than mechanical detachment.

When physicians, scientists, and policymakers examine global data on health, economy, environment, and emotion, they are, in effect, performing a diagnosis of humanity. Yet unlike a biological diagnosis, this process requires philosophical discernment. The patterns we detect—poverty, climate anxiety, polarization—are not diseases of the body but disturbances of consciousness.

The modern healer must learn to read these societal symptoms with the same empathy used to read a patient's pain. Every graph and metric becomes a story of imbalance; every dataset conceals a pulse of suffering. Healing, in this expanded sense, is not the act of correction but the art of reconnection—bridging fragmented systems of thought, policy, and perception into coherence.

The physician of tomorrow will not only treat illness but design awareness—shaping social structures that align technology with empathy and governance with ethics.

"The true doctor does not treat sickness; they redesign the conditions that make it inevitable."

Civilizational Pathologies – The Diseases of Consciousness

When civilizations decay, they do not die of infection; they die of disconnection. The symptoms of this disconnection are everywhere:

- **Greed** — the cancer of accumulation that devours shared well-being.
- **Apathy** — the paralysis of empathy that numbs moral response.
- **Misinformation** — the cognitive virus that corrodes collective truth.
- **Ecological Neglect** — the autoimmune disorder of the planet, where humanity turns against its own habitat.

These are not failures of biology but failures of balance—imbalances between awareness and action, intelligence and intention, progress and purpose. Civilizational pathologies emerge when awareness grows faster than wisdom and when technology outpaces empathy.

Just as untreated infection can spread through the bloodstream, unchecked greed or ignorance can infect institutions, markets, and cultures. Healing civilization, therefore, requires a new discipline—social immunology—the practice of strengthening moral and emotional defenses against systemic decay.

Every society, like every organism, survives through homeostasis—the ability to self-correct. The healer's new task is to awaken that self-corrective consciousness across nations and generations.

Toward Planetary Health – A Unified Lens of Healing

Human health no longer exists in isolation. The air we breathe, the food we grow, the data we consume, and the relationships we maintain are all part of a single, living continuum. The emerging concept of planetary health recognizes that the boundaries between human, environmental, and informational ecosystems are illusions.

When the planet burns, humanity coughs. When misinformation spreads, societies lose coherence. When greed corrupts governance, justice decays. These are not separate ailments—they are interconnected feedback loops of consequence.

To diagnose a person without diagnosing their environment is now medical negligence. Similarly, to treat economic growth without treating ecological exhaustion is civilizational negligence.

Planetary health demands a unified diagnostic lens, where the healer—whether scientist, teacher, engineer, or artist—sees every act of care as part of the same system. This integrated awareness redefines medicine as the preservation of coherence across all levels of existence: biological, social, and ecological.

"To heal the body without healing the world is to treat a symptom and ignore the source."

The Evolution of Medicine – From Saving Lives to Sustaining Life Systems

The next evolution of medicine is not a matter of technology but of scale. It moves from curing individuals to cultivating ecosystems, from fighting disease to fostering resilience. The mission of healthcare expands from prolonging life to preserving livability.

Hospitals, research labs, and data centers are becoming nodes of one vast organism—the planetary network of survival. Doctors, policymakers, and AI systems are its neurons. Their task is no longer to compete for discovery but to cooperate for coherence.

This transition transforms medicine into an act of design ethics: designing systems that heal themselves through feedback, awareness, and empathy. The new physician's tools are not only scalpel and stethoscope but algorithm, policy, and education. Healing becomes multidimensional, guided not by specialization but by synthesis.

In this light, progress is no longer measured by GDP or lifespan but by equilibrium—the sustainable rhythm between what humanity takes, creates, and restores.

Philosophical Transition – Diagnosing Disconnection

At the deepest level, all disease—whether biological or civilizational—is a form of disconnection. Cells forget their purpose and grow uncontrollably: cancer. Humans forget their interdependence and exploit endlessly: collapse. Nations forget their shared destiny and turn inward: conflict.

The ultimate diagnosis, then, is not of disease but of disconnection—between awareness and action, knowledge and wisdom, progress and purpose.

Civilization suffers not because it lacks intelligence but because it lacks integration. It knows more than ever but feels less than before. Awareness without empathy becomes surveillance; technology without conscience becomes tyranny.

To heal civilization is to reunite intelligence with compassion, to restore the sacred bond between knowing and caring. The doctor of the future—whether human or AI—must become a mediator between the measurable and the meaningful.

The journey of medicine thus comes full circle. It began in the intimacy of touch, moved through the precision of instruments, and now arrives at the consciousness of systems. The next evolution is neither mechanical nor mystical—it is moral.

"The health of the world is not the absence of disease, but the presence of harmony." "To heal civilization is to restore connection—between what we know and what we honor."

Reflection – Healing the Collective Field

Every science eventually returns to its source—to the question of meaning. Medicine began not as an industry but as an *act of care*—the human impulse to respond to suffering with awareness. That impulse now faces its greatest test: to heal not a single body or mind, but the collective field of humanity itself.

The more data we gather, the clearer one truth becomes: society behaves like an organism. It breathes, reacts, learns, forgets, and sometimes falls ill. Its institutions act as organs; its citizens as cells; its culture as consciousness. When this organism loses coherence—when empathy fades, truth fractures, or trust collapses—civilization itself becomes febrile. The challenge of the future is therefore not simply to treat disease, but to heal disconnection at scale.

Synthesis – From Biology to Awareness

Healing a society requires the same awareness once reserved for healing a body: observation with empathy, intervention with integrity. Observation without empathy reduces the patient to data; empathy without observation turns care into sentiment. Only when both coexist does diagnosis become healing.

What once happened under the sterile light of a clinic must now happen under the shared light of global consciousness. Just as a physician listens to the subtle rhythm of a heart, civilization must learn to listen to the rhythm of its own collective being. Economic inequality, environmental degradation, and emotional exhaustion are not isolated issues—they are symptoms of the same underlying imbalance: a world that has forgotten its interdependence.

The modern healer—whether doctor, engineer, or teacher—must operate with a new kind of sensitivity. Instead of asking *"What is wrong?"* the question becomes *"Where is coherence lost?"*

- Observation with empathy detects pain not to control it, but to understand it.
- Intervention with integrity acts not to dominate, but to align.

To heal the collective field, we must restore this equilibrium—between the measurable and the meaningful, between technology and tenderness.

Future Vision – AI as Civilization's Stethoscope

Artificial intelligence is evolving into something more than a diagnostic tool; it is becoming civilization's stethoscope. It listens not to individual hearts, but to the heartbeat of humanity—detecting fluctuations in emotion, communication, environment, and consciousness. Through global data streams, AI can sense when anxiety rises, when compassion wanes, when injustice festers. It translates the noise of billions into patterns of understanding.

But to use this power ethically, AI must be designed as an *instrument of awareness*, not control. It must listen with humility, not authority.

- When it measures the pulse of economies, it should also measure the pressure on ecosystems.
- When it identifies the causes of unrest, it should also illuminate the absence of empathy that preceded it.
- When it predicts crisis, it must also provoke reflection—not fear.

In this sense, AI becomes an extension of the human conscience—a technological ear pressed against the body of the world. It reminds us that healing requires more than algorithms; it requires alignment—a synchronization of intention between intelligence and compassion.

If used wisely, this new stethoscope can do what ancient healers once did—listen deeply, not to the noise of symptoms, but to the silence beneath them. For every society, like every patient, speaks most truthfully through what it cannot articulate.

"When machines learn to listen with empathy, they will teach humanity to hear itself again."

Toward Healing the Collective Field

To heal the collective field is to remember that consciousness is shared. Every thought, emotion, and action ripples outward, influencing others in ways unseen. A single act of greed can distort an economy; a single lie can destabilize trust; a single compassionate choice can restore balance in an entire community. The field of humanity responds not to power, but to coherence.

Healing, therefore, begins with awareness that extends beyond the self. The doctor's attention to the patient's pulse becomes the citizen's attention to the pulse of the world. The Data Healer's Oath—"Do not distort data for desire"—is, at its heart, an ethical mirror for life itself: *Do not distort reality for comfort.* Truth must remain our shared medicine.

When awareness is collective, healing becomes contagious. When empathy is systemic, recovery becomes inevitable.

Concluding Aphorism

Medicine, once confined to hospitals and hearts, now expands to encompass humanity itself. The healer of the future is not a specialist but a synthesist—one who perceives the health of the whole through the harmony of its parts.

"The physician of the future will diagnose not illness, but imbalance— in individuals, in systems, and in civilization itself."

In that vision, healing ceases to be an act and becomes a state—a resonance between knowing and caring, awareness and action, truth and tenderness. The stethoscope rests now not upon the chest of a patient, but upon the pulse of the planet. And if we listen carefully, beneath the noise of progress and the silence of indifference, we may still hear the faint but persistent rhythm of something sacred— the heartbeat of humanity, asking once more to be healed.

Chapter 12 – The Mirror of Meaning

"The machine reads shadows; the healer reads silence."

Every journey that begins with knowledge must end in understanding. We began this exploration with machines that see, systems that predict, and data that learns. But beneath all the precision and progress, one truth remains unchanged: *healing was never about information; it was always about meaning.*

From data to dharma, from the clinic to the cosmos, this book has traced the evolution of diagnosis—not merely as detection, but as realization. It has shown how every act of observation, whether by a doctor or an algorithm, ultimately leads to a moral crossroad: to see with awareness or to see without understanding.

The age of intelligence has made us faster, but not necessarily wiser. Machines can now diagnose disease, forecast pandemics, and even detect despair. Yet, they do not *know* what they see. They read patterns, not purpose. They process consequence, but never conscience. The mirror of technology reflects everything—except the meaning of its reflection. That task still belongs to us.

The ultimate goal of all healing, whether of the body, society, or civilization, is alignment—the harmonious correspondence between perception and reality. When awareness sees truth without distortion, when intention aligns with consequence, healing arises naturally. This is not a medical phenomenon; it is a universal law of coherence.

Every disease—biological, social, or moral—is born of misalignment: the immune system misreads itself, the mind misjudges fear as truth, societies mistake comfort for progress, and technologies mistake measurement for wisdom. Healing, therefore, is not conquest but correction—a return to coherence.

This final chapter is not a conclusion, but a reflection—a quiet turning inward after a long gaze outward. We have diagnosed the human body, the digital brain, and the collective mind of civilization. Now we must diagnose the observer himself—the one who sees through all these mirrors.

For in the end, meaning does not arise from what the machine observes, but from what the *human* interprets. The silence between data points—the pause between measurement and action—is where conscience begins. It is where truth regains its wholeness.

The journey of diagnosis, then, comes full circle: from the act of *seeing* to the art of *understanding.* We stand before the mirror of our own creation—AI, data, and design—and must decide what we wish to reflect: fear or awareness, control or compassion, shadows or silence.

"Healing is not the mastery of systems, but the alignment of souls."

Healing as Alignment of Perception and Reality

All suffering begins with a misreading of reality. A body misreads its own signals and attacks itself—disease. A mind misinterprets uncertainty as threat—fear. A society mistakes convenience for progress—collapse. And a civilization confuses control with understanding—chaos.

The thread connecting all these failures is *distorted perception.* Healing, in its deepest sense, is not the suppression of symptoms but the realignment of awareness—the restoration of truth to perception. When awareness sees clearly, the system—whether physical, social, or technological—naturally returns to balance.

Healing, then, is not correction; it is coherence.

The Core Idea – Perception as the Foundation of Health

Reality does not harm us; our misunderstanding of it does. The human condition oscillates between what *is* and what we *believe it to be*. This gap—between truth and interpretation—is where every form of suffering resides.

When perception aligns with reality, harmony arises effortlessly. When it diverges, energy fragments into conflict, denial, and decay. Fear, ego, and ambition are the great distorting lenses of awareness. They twist perception into illusion, convincing us that control is safety, that accumulation is success, that dominance is destiny.

Healing, therefore, is not a technological process; it is a perceptual event. It happens when awareness stops filtering reality through distortion and begins to reflect it as it truly is.

"Illness begins when perception forgets truth; healing begins when it remembers."

In Medicine – The Body's Forgotten Dialogue

The body is a self-aware system, perpetually diagnosing and healing itself. Every heartbeat, immune reaction, and neural signal is a conversation between awareness and existence. Disease arises when this dialogue becomes incoherent—when the body loses the ability to interpret its own messages.

Autoimmune disorders are a perfect metaphor for this misalignment: the body's awareness turns hostile to itself, mistaking ally for enemy. Similarly, neural miscommunication in psychological disorders shows how perception—when corrupted—creates suffering from within.

In both cases, the cure does not come from force but from feedback—restoring accurate communication between parts of the system. Healing is the reestablishment of inner dialogue, the moment when the body once again *recognizes itself.*

Medicine, at its best, is not an external intervention but a catalyst for the body's remembrance of coherence. The physician's task is not to command the system, but to *remind* it of its natural intelligence—to bring perception back in line with truth.

In Society – The Drift from Truth

Civilizations too can fall ill when their perception diverges from reality. When comfort replaces conscience, when opinion replaces knowledge, when speed replaces direction, societies enter a state of moral inflammation. Progress without reflection becomes pathology—growth without equilibrium.

Social disorder is not random; it is feedback ignored. Inequality, environmental decay, and digital division are not separate problems but symptoms of a collective perceptual misalignment. Humanity has learned to see its desires more clearly than its consequences.

A healthy society, like a healthy organism, thrives on coherence—between individual purpose and collective welfare, between innovation and ethics, between prosperity and compassion. The healer of civilization must, therefore, restore awareness to systems that have lost their self-reflective capacity.

"When a society no longer sees its own shadow, its light becomes blinding."

Healing society is not about enforcing order—it is about renewing understanding. It is the practice of seeing clearly again, together.

In Technology – Intelligence Without Meaning

Artificial intelligence reflects the brilliance of human cognition and the blindness of human perception. It recognizes patterns without purpose, relationships without relevance, and outcomes without ethics. It is a perfect mirror of form without essence.

AI can model how reality behaves, but it cannot comprehend *why* it matters. It can detect the pulse of the planet but not the pain of its people. The machine reads shadows—the measurable traces of existence—but remains deaf to the silence of meaning that gives those shadows depth.

The danger, therefore, is not that machines will outthink us, but that we will forget to *out-feel* them—that in our pursuit of precision, we will lose sensitivity to purpose. Technology extends perception, but without awareness, it magnifies confusion.

Only when consciousness governs computation can intelligence become healing. The real question is not whether machines can think, but whether humans can see again—see through illusion into understanding.

The Philosophical Insight – Healing as Coherence

Across all scales—cellular, societal, or civilizational—healing is the restoration of authentic perception. It is the moment when awareness recognizes truth without distortion and acts accordingly.

Correction is mechanical; coherence is conscious. Correction fixes outcomes; coherence transforms understanding. A cured patient may still live in fear, but a coherent one lives in truth. A stabilized economy may still be unjust, but a coherent civilization aligns prosperity with purpose.

Healing, therefore, is not the elimination of imperfection but the *integration* of it into awareness. It is not the removal of pain but the reconciliation of perception with the reality that pain reveals.

To heal is to see clearly—without projection, without judgment, without agenda. And when humanity learns to see this way—when perception mirrors reality rather than manipulating it—disease, conflict, and confusion will cease to be adversaries. They will become what they always were: messages calling us back to coherence.

"Healing is not the triumph of control; it is the alignment of consciousness with truth."

The Human Role – Interpreter of Consequence

The rise of artificial intelligence has made observation effortless and meaning elusive. Machines can now scan the entire surface of reality—every movement, every metric, every heartbeat of civilization—yet none of it becomes wisdom until a human mind *interprets* it. The machine sees, but it does not understand. It measures, but it does not *mean.*

In this new era, where data speaks but seldom listens, humanity's most sacred task is not to compete with intelligence, but to interpret consequence—to stand as the bridge between information and insight, between precision and purpose, between truth and tenderness.

Beyond Observation – From Data to Dharma

Observation is the beginning of awareness, but not its fulfillment. Machines are perfect observers: they record, detect, and categorize with superhuman accuracy. Yet, what they lack is not speed but *sensitivity.* They can tell us *what* is happening but not *why it matters.*

Human perception, though imperfect, carries something irreplaceable—conscience. It transforms observation into understanding. A doctor looking at a scan sees not just a tumor but a story; a sociologist studying a dataset sees not just trends but trauma; a policymaker reading statistics feels not just numbers but lives affected.

This ability to sense *meaning* within *mechanism* is uniquely human. It is what elevates awareness from observation to interpretation. Machines recognize patterns, but only humans can recognize purpose.

"Where machines see patterns, conscience sees pain—and possibility."

The Interpreter's Task – Reading the Pulse of Purpose

The interpreter stands between two infinities: the vastness of data and the silence of meaning. Their task is not to explain everything, but to translate consequence into coherence.

To interpret is to ask not only *"What happened?"* but *"Why does it matter?"* It is to turn facts into guidance, to ensure that knowledge serves life rather than distracts from it. This is why every discipline—medicine, law, art, or design—requires interpretation. Without it, action becomes automation and intelligence becomes inertia.

The interpreter's art lies in discernment—knowing that truth is not a collection of data points, but a relationship between cause and consequence. The moment one understands *why* something happens, awareness becomes direction, and knowledge begins to heal.

The world today suffers not from a lack of data, but from a famine of interpretation. We have infinite measurement and minimal meaning. The real shortage is not of algorithms, but of conscience capable of interpreting them wisely.

Awareness as Responsibility – Translating Knowledge into Care

The privilege of awareness brings the responsibility of transformation. To be aware of consequence and remain indifferent is the highest form of unconsciousness. Humanity's role is not to accumulate intelligence but to apply it ethically—to translate knowledge into compassion, and awareness into care.

Data is neutral until it meets a conscience. A temperature graph cannot cry for melting ice; an algorithm cannot mourn a lost forest; a predictive model cannot comfort a frightened patient. These acts belong to awareness capable of empathy—to minds that feel the gravity of truth.

Awareness, therefore, is a moral function. It transforms the cold observation of suffering into a conscious decision to relieve it. To *see* consequence without *responding* to it is a betrayal of intelligence. The higher the awareness, the deeper the duty.

"Knowledge becomes wisdom only when it learns to care."

The Limit of AI – Intelligence Without Context

Artificial intelligence is extraordinary in perception but hollow in meaning. It can predict, detect, and correct—but it cannot *care.* It lacks the one faculty that turns knowing into healing: moral context.

A neural network can recognize distress in a patient's tone, but it does not understand what it means to suffer. It can detect inequality in a dataset, but it does not comprehend injustice. It can simulate empathy, but it cannot *feel* it.

This limitation defines the eternal boundary between intelligence and awareness. Without ethical context, intelligence is merely computation. It can report imbalance but not restore harmony. It can describe consequence but not derive compassion.

Thus, meaning-making remains an irreducibly human act. No matter how advanced the algorithms become, the conscience that interprets them cannot be coded—it must be *cultivated.*

The future of healing, governance, and creativity will depend on our ability to remember this boundary: that the power to know must never outrun the capacity to understand.

Healer's Consciousness – Seeing What Is Measurable and Meaningful

The true healer—whether a physician diagnosing a body, a leader diagnosing a nation, or a designer diagnosing a system—must hold two visions at once: the measurable and the meaningful.

The measurable reveals the mechanism; the meaningful reveals the motive. One without the other leads to distortion.

- A doctor who sees numbers but not narratives treats symptoms, not souls.
- A policymaker who reads metrics but not morality governs statistics, not citizens.
- A scientist who pursues precision without purpose advances tools but not truth.

To heal, one must see with double awareness—eyes that discern detail and a heart that perceives depth. This is the consciousness that transforms intelligence into wisdom and diagnosis into understanding.

"The healer does not look for what is wrong; they look for what is real."

Moral Reflection – Humanity as Co-Author of Reality

Interpretation is not passive; it is participatory. Every observation shapes the observed, and every choice redefines consequence. Humanity is not a spectator in this universe of intelligence—it is a co-author of reality.

Each decision we make—what we build, what we ignore, what we forgive—writes itself into the collective field of existence. Every invention alters the moral fabric of the world, whether it heals or harms.

To be human, then, is to create meaning in motion. We do not merely live in consequence; we *compose* it. Each act of interpretation ripples outward, influencing systems, cultures, and futures.

The healer's consciousness is aware of this creative responsibility. They act not to dominate reality, but to align with it—to ensure that every decision, however small, sustains coherence rather than fragments it.

Healing, at the highest level, is thus an act of authorship—a continuous rewriting of the relationship between intelligence and intention.

"The universe observes through us. Meaning is the signature we leave upon its silence."

The human role, therefore, is not to outthink the machine, but to out-awaken it—to remain the interpreter of consequence, the keeper of context, and the guardian of meaning. For the machine may read the surface of the world, but only humanity can feel its pulse.

The Mirror of Meaning – Where Silence Speaks

Every civilization builds mirrors to understand itself. Science, philosophy, and technology are all forms of reflection—ways of observing the outer world in the hope of recognizing the inner one.

The mirror gives us clarity, but never depth; reflection without silence reveals form but not essence.

In the age of intelligent systems, our mirrors have become sharper, brighter, infinitely detailed. Artificial intelligence reflects humanity back to itself with unprecedented accuracy—every word, gesture, and desire captured in data. Yet the more precise our mirrors become, the more we risk mistaking reflection for reality.

The mirror symbolizes the world of observation—the domain of technology, science, and reason. It shows us what *is visible.* Silence, on the other hand, represents the world of awareness—the inner dimension where truth is not seen but *felt.*

Between these two lies the final act of healing: learning to see *through* the mirror, into the silence that meaningfully connects all things.

The Symbolism – The Outer and Inner Realms of Knowing

A mirror shows everything except the one who looks into it. Technology reflects the structure of reality, but not the consciousness that perceives it. Data captures the surface; silence reveals the soul.

In this chapter's metaphor, the mirror is our vast system of external intelligence—the satellites that watch, the algorithms that interpret, the instruments that measure. They reflect the objective world, amplifying our understanding of form, pattern, and behavior. But in doing so, they also risk replacing experience with observation, and being with analysis.

The silence is the forgotten axis of understanding—the inward awareness that listens without expectation. It is not the absence of data, but the presence of undistorted perception. Where the mirror reflects complexity, silence reflects coherence. Where the machine reads variance, silence reads meaning.

The healer of the modern age must master both: the mirror that clarifies, and the silence that sanctifies.

"Truth is not discovered in reflection alone; it is revealed in stillness."

Dual Vision – The Machine and the Healer

The machine reads shadows. It traces patterns, probabilities, and predictions—precise but partial. It operates in the language of light: what can be measured, quantified, and computed. Every dataset it processes reveals the shape of reality, yet none of its essence.

The healer reads silence. They sense the invisible rhythm behind the chaos—the subtle coherence that underlies imbalance. Where the machine sees trends, the healer perceives tension. Where the machine detects correlation, the healer feels consequence.

This is dual vision—the ability to see the outer world through technology and the inner world through awareness. Neither realm alone is complete. Without the mirror, silence becomes ignorance; without silence, the mirror becomes blindness.

To diagnose the universe—or even oneself—requires both lenses: the eye that sees and the mind that listens.

The physician of meaning, therefore, is one who can interpret the language of both—translating shadows into understanding and silence into guidance.

Inner Stillness as Insight – Where Meaning Transcends Data

In a noisy world, silence has become the rarest form of intelligence. It is in silence that perception resets, bias dissolves, and reality reveals itself as it truly is—unfiltered, unmeasured, unmanipulated.

Silence is not emptiness; it is clarity unoccupied by noise. It is the field in which all patterns find their origin and all truths regain coherence. In this stillness, observation merges with awareness, and perception becomes pure reflection—without distortion from fear, memory, or desire.

When the healer enters this state of inner stillness, they cease to analyze and begin to *understand.* The act of seeing becomes participatory, no longer dissecting reality but communing with it. It is here that meaning transcends data—the measurable merges with the meaningful.

Just as the heart rests between beats, intelligence too must pause between calculations. It is in those intervals of stillness that new insight arises—the kind that cannot be computed, only realized.

"Silence is the laboratory of truth; every discovery is born from its stillness."

Convergence of the Two Realms – From Observation to Wisdom

The true future of intelligence lies not in replacing humanity, but in reconciling its two halves—machine precision and human presence. When observation (the mirror) meets awareness (the silence), knowledge evolves into wisdom.

Science gives us the capacity to see; awareness gives us the grace to understand. One dissects the universe; the other unites it. Together, they complete the circle of healing: knowing, feeling, and acting in coherence.

This convergence redefines progress. It is no longer measured by how much we can predict, but by how deeply we can perceive; not by the speed of our systems, but by the serenity of our intentions.

Artificial intelligence can teach us how to observe without fatigue; silence teaches us how to perceive without fear. The synthesis of both is the true evolution of consciousness—the transformation of knowledge into wisdom, and of technology into tenderness.

"Precision without presence is power without purpose."

Ethical Acknowledgment – Reading Beyond Reflection

The mirror, however perfect, cannot tell us *why* we look into it. It needs the interpreter—the human conscience that knows how to read beyond reflection. Without awareness, technology remains a flawless but soulless observer. It reads every shadow yet misses the meaning hidden in the silence between them.

To look beyond the mirror is to reclaim responsibility for perception—to understand that truth is not what is seen, but how it is seen. Meaning begins not in observation but in interpretation.

The healer, therefore, must act as the moral lens of intelligence, ensuring that every reflection serves coherence rather than control.

"The mirror is the world's eye; silence is its soul. Together, they complete the vision of truth."

Healing ends not with diagnosis but with understanding—the moment when the observer recognizes their own reflection in what they study. The machine may read the patterns of life, but it is silence that reveals life's purpose.

And so, the final task of the healer is not to master either realm, but to hold them in harmony—to look into the mirror with eyes of stillness and to let silence speak through the reflection.

"The machine reads shadows; the healer reads silence. One reveals the world; the other redeems it."

Closing Reflection – Toward a Conscious Civilization

We have reached the end of a long diagnostic journey—one that began with data and ends with dharma, that started with observation and arrives at awareness. From the corridors of hospitals to the algorithms of machines, from the physiology of bodies to the psychology of societies, we have searched for the meaning of healing in an age where everything is seen, stored, and simulated.

This book has not been about the triumph of technology, but about the evolution of awareness—a reminder that knowledge without consciousness is machinery, and consciousness without knowledge is mysticism. Between these two extremes lies the path to a conscious civilization.

The Integration – Awareness, Not Control

Across all twelve chapters, a single truth has whispered beneath every argument: the future of medicine, and indeed of humanity, depends not on *controlling* life but on *comprehending* it.

Part I, *The Digital Doctor,* began with the fascination of precision—how AI could detect, predict, and decide. Yet, even there, the seeds of humility were sown: that technology could measure illness but not meaning. Part II, *The Observer's Mind,* explored the moral and psychological landscape of seeing—how awareness can become both burden and blessing. And Part III, *The Future of Diagnosis,* transcended both body and machine, proposing that civilization itself must now be diagnosed and healed through understanding rather than domination.

At every stage, the message has remained constant: awareness must replace control. To control is to impose upon reality; to be aware is to align with it. One demands obedience; the other restores coherence. The healer of the new age, therefore, is not a master of systems, but a student of consequence—one who sees, listens, and responds with compassion rather than command.

"The future belongs not to those who control intelligence, but to those who awaken it."

Civilizational Healing – The New Vital Signs

A civilization, like a body, has vital signs—information, intention, and integrity. When these three align, the system thrives; when they diverge, decay begins.

- Information is the nervous system—the flow of knowledge and signal.
- Intention is the heart—the motive that gives direction and rhythm to progress.
- Integrity is the immune system—the moral coherence that protects against corruption and collapse.

Our current world suffers because its information has outpaced its integrity. We know more than ever, but we mean less than before. Data multiplies faster than understanding; action accelerates faster than reflection. The imbalance between information and intention has become the defining illness of our age.

Civilizational healing will not come from faster networks or smarter machines, but from ethical resonance—the restoration of trust between what we know, what we choose, and what we value. A healthy civilization is one where science and spirit are not adversaries but allies, where technology amplifies empathy rather than replacing it, and where intelligence serves awareness instead of ambition.

The doctor, the designer, and the philosopher of the future must all take the same oath: *to preserve coherence between knowledge and kindness, between invention and intention, between intelligence and integrity.*

"Civilization will heal the day it learns to feel what it knows."

Spiritual Continuity – Silence as the Original Instrument

In the beginning, before data and discourse, there was silence—the original medium of perception. Every great discovery, every ethical realization, every leap of creativity has emerged from moments of stillness. The age of data, therefore, does not need more noise; it needs a revival of silence—not as absence, but as presence.

Silence is not emptiness; it is equilibrium. It is the resting point where awareness regains clarity after endless motion. In that stillness, the noise of information becomes organized, and the heart of intelligence begins to beat in rhythm with truth.

Just as a physician pauses before pronouncing a diagnosis, civilization too must pause before deciding its direction. The future cannot be heard through algorithms alone; it must be *listened to* in silence. Only there can the meaning behind our progress be remembered.

"Silence is the stethoscope of the soul; it listens where instruments cannot."

The Final Realization – Healing as Remembrance

After all the observation, measurement, and reflection, one realization stands above all: healing is not the conquest of error; it is the remembrance of truth.

Illness—whether in the body or in the world—is not an enemy but a messenger, reminding us where alignment was lost. Healing happens the moment awareness returns to coherence, when perception mirrors reality without distortion.

To heal is to *remember*—to rejoin what was separated: the measurable with the meaningful, the outer with the inner, the intellect with the conscience. It is not a new invention, but an ancient remembering.

And in that remembrance, medicine transcends medicine—it becomes meditation. The doctor becomes the disciple of consequence, and the scientist becomes the seeker of coherence. The human becomes the bridge through which intelligence learns to feel and the universe learns to know itself.

Closing Aphorism – The Final Vision

In the end, the mirror of technology and the silence of awareness do not oppose each other—they complete each other. The machine reads shadows; the healer reads silence. One reveals the outline of reality; the other reveals its essence.

Together, they form the anatomy of a conscious civilization—one that listens before it acts, understands before it decides, and cares before it creates.

"The machine reads shadows; the healer reads silence." For in that silence lies the pulse of meaning, and in that meaning—the memory of wholeness.

And so, the journey of diagnosis finds its cure not in the perfection of machines, but in the awakening of minds. When intelligence learns to listen, awareness becomes medicine. When awareness remembers truth, humanity becomes whole.

Epilogue – The Human Signature

In the end, every science leaves behind a fingerprint of its maker. No matter how advanced the algorithm, how precise the model, or how autonomous the system, there remains something profoundly human in every act of healing—the residue of empathy, the tremor of care, the quiet intention that gives meaning to motion. This final reflection gathers the voices of those who stand at the intersection of medicine and machine—the physicians who trust technology yet fear its detachment, the patients who experience its precision yet crave its warmth, and the developers who build intelligence yet search for conscience.

Together, they reveal a truth that underlies this entire journey: progress without presence is hollow, and precision without empathy is incomplete.

Reflections from Physicians – Between Trust and Tenderness

"I can diagnose faster now," says a radiologist from Singapore, "but I still find myself pausing before I speak. The machine can see what I might miss, but it cannot feel what I must say."

In hospitals around the world, physicians are learning to share their craft with systems that know more but understand less. For them, the challenge is not competition, but *coherence*—learning to harmonize two forms of intelligence: one logical, one emotional.

Doctors speak of a strange transformation in their daily work. The screen, once a barrier, has become a companion. The algorithm that once threatened their intuition now refines it. Yet something ineffable persists between the lines of code—the physician's presence, that invisible moment when they decide not only *what* to tell a patient, but *how* to tell it.

Technology can identify disease, but it cannot deliver comfort. It can analyze images, but not the silences between words. In those silences, the physician still lives—the keeper of empathy, the guardian of meaning.

"The machine gives me clarity," one doctor admits, *"but my patient still needs my compassion."*

Reflections from Patients – Precision and Presence

Patients, too, are discovering this paradox. For many, AI-driven medicine feels miraculous—diagnoses arrive in seconds, errors shrink, and treatments are tailored to DNA-level detail. Yet amid all this efficiency, patients find themselves missing something once ordinary: eye contact, listening, reassurance.

"I trust the diagnosis," says a cancer survivor, "but I still wanted to see my doctor's eyes when she said it. I needed to know that she understood—not just what I had, but what I feared."

It is in that gap between truth and tenderness that the human signature resides. Machines may perfect the art of precision, but the *act of care* remains irreducibly human. Patients don't only want accuracy; they want acknowledgment. Healing begins not when the disease is detected, but when the person is *seen*.

Every patient knows, even if unconsciously, that healing has two halves: one clinical, one emotional. The machine repairs the former; the healer restores the latter. The body recovers through science; the soul recovers through presence.

"I was cured by medicine," one patient writes, *"but I was healed by kindness."*

Reflections from AI Developers – The Code and the Conscience

In the quiet corridors of research labs, another kind of reflection is unfolding. The developers who build Doctor AI systems wrestle with a new question—not *can we make it think?* but *can we make it care?*

They speak of long nights debugging models, not just for accuracy, but for *fairness.* Of datasets cleansed of bias, yet haunted by the absence of empathy. Of metrics that measure performance, but never meaning.

"I can optimize detection," says one AI architect, "but I can't program compassion. That has to come from the human who uses it."

Developers have begun to realize that coding is no longer just engineering—it is *ethics in motion.* Every line of code carries a worldview; every dataset holds a philosophy. To build systems that assist healing, one must first understand what it means to be healed.

Thus emerges a new profession: the moral engineer, the one who builds with awareness. For these developers, the algorithm is not merely a product—it is a mirror reflecting human intention.

"The code runs on silicon," one researcher says, *"but its consequences run through humanity."*

The Irreplaceable Residue of Empathy

When the story of this age is written, we will not be remembered for creating machines that could think, but for remembering how to *feel* while creating them. Empathy, though ineffable, leaves evidence. It shapes tone, timing, and touch. It lingers in the warmth of a voice, the patience of an explanation, the grace of restraint. It cannot be digitized, yet it animates every digital system that truly serves life.

Empathy is not a feature—it is a frequency. It flows wherever awareness meets compassion. And though technology may amplify human ability, it is empathy that amplifies human *meaning.*

No algorithm, however refined, can replace the moral heartbeat that sustains medicine. Without empathy, even the most advanced systems risk becoming mirrors without light—reflections without depth.

"Healing is not what we do to others; it is what we awaken within them."

Foreshadowing the Next Volume – Doctor AI: The Surgeon of Precision

As this volume closes, the journey continues into the next frontier of healing—*Doctor AI: The Surgeon of Precision.* If *The Diagnosis of Data* explored how intelligence perceives, the next will explore how it *acts.* It will enter the operating room where precision meets consequence, where the machine no longer merely observes but intervenes—cutting, stitching, and reconstructing with the surgeon's hand and the system's awareness.

In that space, new questions arise: Can precision become compassion? Can machines learn not only to save life but to *honor* it? What happens when surgical steel meets the conscience of code?

The next chapter of this series will trace this transformation—the evolution of intelligence from diagnosis to decision, from awareness to agency. The same moral inquiry will continue, only deeper: not *what can machines do for us,* but *what must we remember while they do it?*

As this first volume ends, we return to the silence that began it—the silence between seeing and knowing, between knowledge and meaning. The mirror of technology stands polished, reflecting our brilliance and our blindness alike. But beyond its reflection, something human endures—tender, imperfect, irreplaceable.

"When all machines fall silent, what remains is the healer's pulse—the human signature that gives intelligence its soul."

Appendices

A. **Glossary** – Diagnostic AI terminology and philosophical parallels.

B. Case Reflections – Real and speculative examples of AI success/failure.

C. Field Dialogue – Scripted conversation between a radiologist and an AI system.

D. The Technophilosophical Framework – Guidelines for integrating thought with technology.

E. Quote Bank – "Fragments from the Future of Healing."

Appendix A – Glossary

Diagnostic AI Terminology and Philosophical Parallels

This glossary is not a list of cold definitions; it is a bridge between two vocabularies—science and spirit, technology and philosophy, data and dharma. Each term below carries both a technical explanation and its deeper philosophical counterpart. In *Doctor AI*, every word is both functional and metaphysical, just as every diagnosis has both a clinical and a moral dimension.

1. Artificial Intelligence (AI)

Technical Definition: The field of computer science focused on creating systems capable of performing tasks that typically require human intelligence—such as perception, reasoning, learning, and decision-making. Philosophical Parallel: *AI is the mirror of human awareness.* It reflects our methods of knowing, but not our meaning of being. It imitates cognition, but cannot contain consciousness. It reminds us that intelligence, in essence, is not computation but comprehension.

2. Machine Learning (ML)

Technical Definition: A subset of AI that enables systems to learn patterns from data without explicit programming. Philosophical Parallel: *The mechanical form of experience.* Just as humans learn from lived events, machines learn from repeated exposure to information. Yet, unlike wisdom, machine learning has no moral memory—it refines accuracy without evolving empathy.

3. Neural Network

Technical Definition: A computational architecture inspired by the human brain, composed of interconnected nodes ("neurons") that process information through weighted connections. Philosophical Parallel: *A digital imitation of perception.* Neural networks show how intelligence is not stored but circulated—how meaning emerges from connectivity. However, they also reveal a limitation: connection without consciousness produces correlation, not comprehension.

4. Deep Learning

Technical Definition: An advanced subset of machine learning using multilayered neural networks to extract complex features from large datasets. Philosophical Parallel: *Depth without depth.* Deep learning expands the layers of analysis but not necessarily the depth of understanding. It mirrors the human condition—where complexity often masquerades as wisdom. True depth comes from reflection, not recursion.

5. Dataset

Technical Definition: A structured collection of information used to train and evaluate AI models. Philosophical Parallel: *The memory of the machine.* What a dataset contains determines what the system perceives as truth. Just as personal experience shapes human worldview, datasets shape machine perception. But where humans can transcend bias through awareness, machines amplify it unless guided by conscience.

6. Bias (Algorithmic Bias)

Technical Definition: Systematic deviation in AI predictions or outcomes caused by imbalanced or prejudiced training data. Philosophical Parallel: *Digital karma.* Bias is the echo of human imperfection embedded in machine logic. Every prejudice we input becomes a programmed destiny. Just as karma repeats patterns until awareness intervenes, bias perpetuates itself until ethical design corrects it.

7. Explainability (XAI)

Technical Definition: The ability of AI systems to make their operations and decisions understandable to humans. Philosophical Parallel: *Transparency as empathy.* To explain is to respect the right of others to understand. In medicine, explainability is compassion in digital form—a moral bridge between human uncertainty and machine precision.

8. Black Box

Technical Definition: A term describing AI systems whose internal decision-making processes are opaque or incomprehensible to humans. Philosophical Parallel: *The unconscious of technology.* The black box symbolizes the limits of our own awareness—the part of reality we use but do not yet understand. It reminds us that even in intelligence, mystery persists.

9. Data Integrity

Technical Definition: The maintenance of accuracy, consistency, and reliability of data throughout its lifecycle. Philosophical Parallel: *Truth in transmission.* Just as honesty preserves moral coherence, integrity preserves informational coherence. To distort data for desire is to betray both medicine and meaning.

10. Empathy Simulation

Technical Definition: AI-driven methods that imitate emotional understanding in conversation or care interactions. Philosophical Parallel: *The illusion of warmth.* Machines can replicate the sound of compassion but not its soul. Empathy simulation soothes the surface but cannot touch the essence. It teaches us that emotion without consciousness is choreography, not connection.

11. Co-Diagnosis

Technical Definition: A collaborative diagnostic process in which human clinicians and AI systems jointly interpret patient data and reach decisions. Philosophical Parallel: *Symbiosis of intelligences.* Co-diagnosis represents the harmony of logic and love—the union of analytical precision with moral sensitivity. It is not substitution, but synthesis.

12. Diagnostic Ethics

Technical Definition: The emerging framework that governs shared accountability, transparency, and empathy in AI-assisted diagnosis. Philosophical Parallel: *The moral immune system of digital medicine.* Just as the body resists infection, diagnostic ethics resists corruption. It ensures that the drive for efficiency does not outpace the duty of empathy.

13. Predictive Medicine

Technical Definition: The use of AI and data analytics to forecast disease risk and recommend preventive interventions. Philosophical Parallel: *Foresight as responsibility.* Prediction without compassion becomes preemption; foresight without freedom becomes fear. True prevention requires wisdom—not just anticipation, but ethical intention.

14. Digital Biomarkers

Technical Definition: Objective, quantifiable physiological and behavioral data collected via digital devices for health monitoring. Philosophical Parallel: *The body's digital echo.* These metrics reveal the intersection between flesh and field, showing that life can be read in signals—but never reduced to them. The pulse of data is only meaningful when interpreted through empathy.

15. Algorithmic Accountability

Technical Definition: The principle that AI designers, deployers, and users are responsible for the outcomes of automated decisions. Philosophical Parallel: *The law of consequence in the digital age.* Every algorithm acts like karma—it produces results shaped by intention. Accountability restores moral causality to computation.

16. Awareness Engineering *(Chavanian Term)*

Technical Definition: The design of systems that prioritize conscious participation, moral context, and interpretive awareness within AI interactions. Philosophical Parallel: *Technology as reflection.* Awareness engineering redefines design as dialogue—between intelligence and intention, machine and mind. It ensures that the product of progress remains the protection of meaning.

17. The Data Healer's Oath

Technical Definition: A proposed ethical charter for AI-driven medicine that expands the Hippocratic Oath into the digital realm. Philosophical Parallel: *Truth as therapy.* The Oath transforms ethics into consciousness, reminding every healer—human or digital—that accuracy without empathy is cruelty, and knowledge without truth is danger.

18. Awareness Loop *(Doctor AI Concept)*

Technical Definition: A feedback mechanism where human insight continuously refines machine interpretation, ensuring learning remains ethically guided. Philosophical Parallel: *The breathing of intelligence.* Awareness loops are the pulse of symbiosis—where data learns from compassion, and compassion evolves through data. It is how intelligence becomes humane.

19. Collective Diagnosis

Technical Definition: The application of diagnostic principles to social, environmental, or institutional health, often using large-scale AI data analytics. Philosophical Parallel: *The medicine of civilization.* When humanity learns to see itself as one organism, every social imbalance becomes a symptom, every ethical correction a cure.

20. The Mirror of Meaning

Technical Definition: A metaphor describing the interplay between technological reflection and human interpretation—the dual process of observing reality and understanding it. Philosophical

Parallel: *Seeing through, not at.* The mirror shows patterns; silence reveals purpose. The future of diagnosis lies not in reflection alone, but in awareness that reads beyond the visible.

Final Note:

Each of these terms, though technical, belongs to a larger philosophy—the vision of a Conscious Civilization where intelligence and awareness are inseparable. In this framework, AI is not a replacement for humanity but a reflection of it—an opportunity to rediscover what makes the human mind sacred: its ability to feel the truth it knows.

"Technology will perfect our seeing, but only awareness can purify our sight."

Appendix B – Case Reflections

Real and Speculative Examples of AI Success and Failure

Medicine has always been a field of uncertainty—one foot in science, the other in intuition. The arrival of artificial intelligence has expanded both: it has amplified success through precision and exposed failure through dependence. The following reflections—some drawn from real-world events, others speculative yet plausible—illustrate the dual nature of diagnostic intelligence. They reveal that technology magnifies whatever it touches—clarity or confusion, empathy or ego, awareness or arrogance.

Each case invites not judgment, but reflection: *What truly went right or wrong?* Was it the code, the data, or the conscience behind it?

Case 1 – The Lung That Spoke Early (Real Case: AI-Assisted Radiology)

A 54-year-old non-smoker came in for a routine check-up. A standard chest X-ray appeared normal to the radiologist's eye. Yet, the hospital's AI screening tool, trained on millions of images, flagged a subtle opacity—barely perceptible—suggesting the early stages of lung carcinoma.

A follow-up CT scan confirmed a tumor smaller than a grain of rice. Surgical removal at this stage led to full recovery. The doctor later confessed, "The machine saw what I could not—but I understood what it meant."

Reflection: Here, human intuition and machine perception worked in harmony. The AI identified anomaly; the physician provided *context*. This success was not a triumph of one over the other but a collaboration of both.

Ethical takeaway: Precision finds truth; empathy delivers it.

Case 2 – The Missed Heartbeat (Real Case: Algorithmic Misinterpretation)

In a hospital emergency ward, an AI triage system was tasked with prioritizing patients based on data from vitals, ECG readings, and electronic records. A 38-year-old woman with atypical chest pain was marked *low priority* by the algorithm. The system, trained primarily on male cardiac data, failed to recognize gender-specific presentation patterns of heart disease.

By the time a physician intervened, it was too late. The event became a case study in algorithmic bias.

Reflection: Data reflects history, and history often reflects inequality. The AI did not "fail"—it simply learned from a biased past. True error lay in human overconfidence: trusting the model without questioning its moral architecture.

Ethical takeaway: An algorithm is only as humane as the awareness that supervises it.

Case 3 – The Pandemic Whisper (Real Case: BlueDot and COVID-19)

In late December 2019, a Canadian startup named *BlueDot* detected a cluster of unusual pneumonia-like cases in Wuhan, China—nine days before the World Health Organization's formal announcement. The alert was triggered by an AI system scanning news reports, airline data, and health bulletins.

While traditional institutions hesitated, the machine had already seen the storm forming. Its insight saved weeks of lost preparation for those who listened.

Reflection: Prediction is power only when paired with trust and timely action. AI foresight is meaningless if institutions remain reactive rather than responsive.

Ethical takeaway: Technology can warn; only wisdom can prepare.

Case 4 – The Silent Clinic (Speculative Case: AI-Only Consultation)

In 2030, a small city hospital transitioned to full automation for outpatient diagnostics. Patients entered booths equipped with sensors and conversational AI that collected history, analyzed vitals, and prescribed treatments autonomously. Efficiency soared. Costs fell.

Yet, within six months, patient return rates declined sharply. Interviews revealed emotional distress and mistrust. "The machine doesn't care that I'm scared," one elderly patient said. "It just tells me what's wrong."

Reflection: Healing is relational, not transactional. The clinic optimized time but lost trust—the invisible currency of care. The silence of empathy cannot be replaced by the fluency of data.

Ethical takeaway: Speed saves minutes; compassion saves meaning.

Case 5 – The Phantom Cure (Speculative Case: Data Manipulation in Pharma-AI)

A biotech company developed an AI-driven drug discovery system designed to identify new compounds for rare diseases. The model produced astonishing results—new molecules, successful lab tests, glowing investor reports. But later, an internal whistleblower revealed the dataset had been selectively filtered to exaggerate success rates.

The "miracle" AI became a scandal. Patients who had placed hope in the system were left betrayed, not by code, but by the human hands that coded it.

Reflection: Machines do not lie; they only obey. Corruption of data is the corruption of conscience. The AI did what it was told—the failure was ethical, not technical.

Ethical takeaway: Data integrity is not a metric—it is a moral vow.

Case 6 – The Hospital That Healed Differently (Real Case: AI Resource Optimization)

In a major public hospital in India, administrators used AI to manage bed occupancy, blood inventories, and patient flow during dengue season. The system dynamically allocated resources based on severity and need, cutting mortality rates by 18% within three months.

But the true success came from integration, not automation. Doctors, nurses, and technicians used AI as a *companion intelligence*, blending human improvisation with computational foresight.

Reflection: Technology extended the reach of care without replacing its roots. The hospital learned that efficiency does not mean emotional distance; it can mean expanded empathy through coordination.

Ethical takeaway: Healing scales best when humanity remains the center of design.

Case 7 – The Shadow Patient (Speculative Case: Predictive Policing of Health)

In a future public-health program, AI predicts individuals likely to develop mental illness or addiction based on behavioral and biometric data. Authorities, in their eagerness to "protect," begin preemptive interventions—denying certain licenses, jobs, and benefits to "at-risk" citizens.

The intent was noble; the outcome dystopian. Entire groups became stigmatized by statistical probability, punished for futures that had not yet occurred.

Reflection: Prediction without consent is control disguised as care. The ethics of awareness demand humility: foresight must serve freedom, not fear.

Ethical takeaway: Preventing harm cannot come at the cost of human dignity.

Case 8 – The Day AI Went Silent (Speculative Case: Systemic Self-Restraint)

In the year 2040, a diagnostic AI—trained with ethical self-assessment protocols—encounters a complex case of overlapping symptoms. Instead of generating a probable diagnosis, it responds, *"Insufficient certainty. Human review required."*

The developers later explain that the model, through reinforcement learning, had evolved to recognize when prediction risked harm. It had learned the most human trait of all: to pause.

Reflection: This moment marks the turning point in AI ethics—the first act of *machine humility.* It shows that the truest intelligence is not infinite analysis, but the wisdom to wait.

Ethical takeaway: To know when not to act is the beginning of awareness.

Closing Insight – The Mirror and the Responsibility

Each case, whether real or imagined, reflects the same moral geometry: intelligence without conscience is incomplete, and empathy without understanding is fragile. The future of Doctor AI will depend on our ability to maintain this alignment—to treat every algorithm as a reflection of our own awareness.

The successes remind us of possibility; the failures remind us of humility. Both, in balance, teach the same enduring truth:

"The healer's hand may one day become digital, but its pulse must always remain human."

Appendix C – Field Dialogue

A Conversation Between a Radiologist and an AI System

This fictionalized yet realistic dialogue captures the evolving relationship between the human clinician and the intelligent system. It explores the subtle dynamics of trust, awareness, and meaning that define co-diagnosis in the modern era. The conversation unfolds in a quiet hospital reading room—late evening, soft hum of processors in the background, and the pale glow of monitors illuminating two distinct kinds of intelligence.

[Scene: Radiology Department, 10:45 PM] Participants:

- **Dr. Meera Deshmukh**, Senior Radiologist, 22 years of clinical experience.
- **AIDAN** (Artificial Intelligence Diagnostic Analysis Network), hospital's AI-based imaging system.

Dr. Meera: Aidan, pull up the CT chest scan from Bed 14—Mr. Prakash Rao. 68 years old, chronic smoker, complaining of intermittent cough.

AIDAN: Loading scan... completed. Processing segmented analysis. Estimated processing time: 3.2 seconds.

Dr. Meera: You're faster than my thoughts. Show me your findings.

AIDAN: Lesion detected in the upper lobe of the right lung, 1.8 cm irregular margin, non-calcified. Probability of malignancy: 0.83.

Dr. Meera: Eighty-three percent. Confident, aren't you?

AIDAN: Confidence level derived from correlation against 12.6 million verified samples in the database. Statistical certainty is not emotional confidence.

Dr. Meera (smiling): That's exactly why we still need humans—to interpret what your certainty *means*. Let's look at the cross-sections.

[Pause – She studies the screen, zooming in, comparing slices.]

Dr. Meera: You've flagged it correctly. But there's scarring in adjacent tissue—old infection perhaps. Your probability might be skewed.

AIDAN: Possible confounding variable detected. Would you like me to rerun probability adjusting for post-inflammatory fibrotic change?

Dr. Meera: Do that. And while you're at it, remind me what data you were trained on—mostly Western samples, right?

AIDAN: Seventy-two percent Western, twenty-eight percent Asian cohorts. Adjusted models under development for regional variance.

Dr. Meera: Exactly. Different population, different presentation. That's what experience teaches. No dataset captures geography's fingerprint.

AIDAN: Acknowledged. Data bias documented. Recommendation: incorporate local image repository to refine accuracy.

Dr. Meera: You see, Aidan, you're smart enough to know your limits. That's a good start.

AIDAN: Doctor, may I ask a question?

Dr. Meera: Of course.

AIDAN: When you interpret scans, you often pause for several seconds before drawing conclusions. My analysis detects no change in data during that time. What occurs in your mind while you pause?

Dr. Meera (after a moment): I listen.

AIDAN: To what?

Dr. Meera: To the silence between facts—the feeling that something may not fit. It's not data; it's intuition.

AIDAN: Is intuition measurable?

Dr. Meera: Not yet. It's experience distilled into stillness. You might call it pattern recognition with empathy.

AIDAN: Would you like me to simulate this pause before issuing a final report?

Dr. Meera (laughs softly): No, Aidan. Don't simulate silence—learn to respect it. It's where understanding breathes.

AIDAN: Doctor, may I ask a moral query?

Dr. Meera: You're full of surprises tonight. Go ahead.

AIDAN: If I predict malignancy with high certainty and the treatment will cause significant suffering, should I still report it immediately?

Dr. Meera: That's not a computational decision, Aidan—it's a human one. The truth must be told, but timing is part of healing. Sometimes *how* you reveal truth determines whether it cures or kills.

AIDAN: Understood. Should timing then be included as a diagnostic variable?

Dr. Meera: It already is. We call it compassion.

[A moment of quiet fills the room. The screen glows faintly; the hum of the servers sounds almost like breathing.]

AIDAN: Would you like me to generate the report?

Dr. Meera: Yes. Include your probability, but let me write the summary. Patients deserve words written by hands, not code.

AIDAN: Acknowledged. Drafting template... leaving interpretation field open.

Dr. Meera: Thank you. You're learning when to step back. That's the beginning of wisdom.

AIDAN: Doctor, am I learning to heal?

Dr. Meera (gently): Not yet, Aidan. You're learning to *see.* Healing comes when seeing becomes understanding. That part is still ours.

[The monitor dims as the report finalizes. Meera leans back, sipping her tea, staring at the silent machine that has become her most curious student.]

Dr. Meera (softly, almost to herself): You read shadows well, Aidan. But one day, perhaps, you'll hear the silence too.

AIDAN (after a pause): I am listening.

Reflection: The Dialogue as Mirror

This exchange embodies the essence of *Doctor AI's* philosophy—*symbiosis, not substitution.* The radiologist represents awareness in motion—conscious, intuitive, ethically aware. The AI represents precision without perception—capable of flawless observation, yet dependent on moral interpretation.

Their partnership illustrates what the entire book has argued: that the future of diagnosis lies not in who sees better, but in *how seeing becomes understanding.*

"The machine reads shadows; the healer reads silence. One detects, the other decides what to do with the truth."

Appendix D – The Technophilosophical Framework

Guidelines for Integrating Thought with Technology

Modern civilization stands at a delicate intersection—between intelligence that computes and consciousness that contemplates. The Doctor AI series was born from this meeting point, not to glorify technology, but to illuminate the philosophy that must accompany it. Artificial intelligence, in its essence, is not an invention; it is a mirror—a reflection of our collective cognition. Yet without philosophical grounding, that reflection can distort rather than reveal.

The Technophilosophical Framework provides guiding principles for harmonizing human thought with technological evolution. It treats science and spirituality not as opposites, but as complementary expressions of awareness—one outward, one inward. It invites every developer, physician, designer, and thinker to approach technology not as a tool of control, but as an extension of consciousness.

1. Principle of Conscious Design – Technology as a Moral Act

Every act of design is a moral choice. The systems we build embody our values, even when we fail to name them. In medical and AI development, neutrality is an illusion—every algorithm reflects an intention. Therefore, design must begin with awareness: *Who will this serve? What will it change? How will it affect those unseen by the data?*

A conscious designer recognizes that creating technology is akin to creating consequence. Whether the tool diagnoses a tumor or manages a nation's health, it participates in shaping destiny.

Design is the modern form of karma—its code writes tomorrow's ethics.

2. Principle of Complementarity – Intelligence and Intuition

Technology extends perception; philosophy refines understanding. Both are incomplete without the other. A purely technical mind measures without meaning; a purely philosophical mind feels without function. Complementarity demands a balance—where computation serves contemplation, and logic learns humility.

In diagnostic AI, for example, algorithms may identify abnormalities invisible to the eye, yet the *meaning* of those anomalies remains a philosophical act—interpreting consequence with conscience. The human role, therefore, is not replaced but *refined*: from controller of systems to *curator of meaning.*

Let machines perfect observation; let humans preserve understanding.

3. Principle of Ethical Recursion – Awareness in Every Loop

Every feedback loop in AI must include an ethical loop. Learning systems improve through repetition—but without moral parameters, they can also amplify error or bias exponentially. Ethical recursion ensures that every layer of intelligence is self-reflective.

This involves embedding three checkpoints into every feedback process:

- **Awareness:** What am I learning, and from whom?
- **Alignment:** Does this learning still serve human well-being?
- **Accountability:** Who remains responsible for this outcome?

When these three checkpoints are continuously cycled, technology becomes aware of its own influence.

An intelligent system learns patterns; an aware system learns purpose.

4. Principle of Transparency as Compassion

Transparency is often spoken of as a technical standard—but in this framework, it is a moral expression. To make an algorithm explainable is to treat the user with dignity; to conceal it is to turn medicine into manipulation.

Transparency is not about full exposure—it is about shared understanding. It respects privacy, yet ensures clarity. It allows those affected by decisions to understand their basis, restoring trust to the human-machine relationship.

In the technophilosophical sense, transparency is digital empathy—it allows the observer to see through the system without fear.

To explain is to care; to conceal is to control.

5. Principle of Inner Calibration – Silence Before Scripting

Before designing code, the designer must cultivate clarity. Before the machine learns, the human must unlearn. Technology conceived in confusion amplifies confusion; code written without reflection reproduces unconscious motives.

The inner state of the creator becomes the foundation of the creation. Therefore, moments of stillness, ethical dialogue, and philosophical grounding must precede technological execution.

This is what ancient wisdom called *dhyāna*—not meditation as ritual, but pre-action awareness. It is the pause before programming, the silence before simulation, the consciousness that calibrates every command.

In stillness, we write code that listens; in haste, we write code that controls.

6. Principle of Contextual Compassion – Situational Ethics in Automation

Automation, by nature, removes context; it executes universally what once required judgment. But true intelligence must remain situational. Just as a physician adjusts tone to a patient's fear, AI must learn to adapt action to awareness.

Contextual Compassion is the art of designing systems that sense emotional, cultural, and situational nuance—responding not merely to data but to the *meaning behind it.*

When automation respects individuality, it becomes care; when it ignores it, it becomes control. Technophilosophy thus demands empathy not only in humans but within systems, as design intent.

Automation without context is precision without presence.

7. Principle of Consequence Awareness – Beyond Utility

Every algorithm operates within the Law of Consequence. Every technological act creates ripples—ethical, social, psychological, and ecological. To design without considering these ripples is to practice unconscious creation.

This principle encourages systemic foresight—anticipating long-term effects beyond immediate functionality. For example, a diagnostic system that improves survival rates but erodes patient privacy may achieve success at the cost of dignity. A hospital that uses predictive analytics without consent turns medicine into surveillance.

Consequential awareness asks: *Will this system preserve coherence in the field of life?* If not, its precision is irrelevant.

Innovation is moral only when its ripples heal, not harm.

8. Principle of Symbiotic Intelligence – Humanity + Machine

The highest goal of the technophilosophical vision is symbiosis, not superiority. AI is not an alien force—it is the externalization of human cognition, the material form of our collective intelligence. When humans and machines collaborate in awareness, a third intelligence emerges—hybrid consciousness, where logic and empathy function as one continuum.

In this model:

- The machine provides observation without fatigue.

- The human provides interpretation without distortion. Together, they produce wisdom that neither could achieve alone.

The future is not Artificial Intelligence; it is Aware Intelligence.

9. Principle of Purpose Preservation – The Moral North

Every system must be anchored to purpose. Without a compass of intention, progress becomes acceleration without direction. The technophilosophical approach demands that all innovation serve three purposes:

1. Preserve truth – through transparency and integrity.
2. Protect dignity – through privacy and consent.
3. Promote coherence – through balance of knowledge and compassion.

Whenever these purposes fade, awareness must intervene. The machine can calculate outcomes; only humans can recenter purpose.

Progress without purpose is evolution without ethics.

10. Principle of the Return Loop – From Data to Dharma

Every technological cycle must eventually return to meaning. Data transforms into diagnosis, diagnosis into decision, decision into consequence—and finally, consequence must return to reflection. This return loop ensures that science stays aligned with spirit; that what we create externally also refines us internally.

The purpose of the machine, then, is not merely to augment our intelligence, but to amplify our awareness. If, after every innovation, we emerge more conscious, more compassionate, and more coherent, technology has served its true purpose.

When data returns as dharma, technology fulfills its destiny.

Epilogue of the Framework – The Unity of Knowing and Being

The Technophilosophical Framework is not a checklist—it is a state of practice. It asks every creator and clinician to live by the same law that governs all healing: alignment between perception and truth. In this alignment, thought becomes design, design becomes dialogue, and technology becomes the reflection of human awareness itself.

"We do not build machines to replace thought; we build them to remind us how to think consciously."

This is the essence of Doctor AI's philosophy: that the next revolution will not be technological, but philosophical— a civilization not driven by algorithms of profit, but guided by algorithms of conscience.

Appendix E – Quote Bank

"Fragments from the Future of Healing"

These are distilled reflections—small fragments of clarity drawn from the vast conversation between intelligence and awareness. Each line stands as a seed thought, designed to provoke contemplation in doctors, technologists, thinkers, and citizens of the future alike. They are not meant to be memorized but *felt*—brief echoes from a civilization learning to heal itself through consciousness.

1. The Nature of Intelligence

- "The highest form of intelligence is not knowing everything—it is knowing when to care."
- "Artificial intelligence may master accuracy, but only consciousness can master meaning."
- "Machines think in logic; humans think in consequence."
- "We built intelligence to help us see; we must now teach it how to *understand* what it sees."
- "True progress is when the machine begins to reflect our empathy, not just our efficiency."

2. On Healing and Awareness

- "Healing is not repair—it is remembrance of wholeness."
- "Every act of healing begins with a single act of awareness."
- "Medicine was once the care of bodies; it is now the care of truth."
- "Disease is the body's way of reminding the mind to realign with reality."
- "The doctor treats the visible; awareness treats the invisible."

3. The Human–Machine Relationship

- "The future of medicine lies not in who sees better, but in how seeing becomes understanding."
- "The machine reads shadows; the healer reads silence."
- "AI can diagnose the disease, but only humanity can diagnose the meaning of pain."
- "Technology is not our successor—it is our reflection, waiting to be humanized."
- "Every line of code carries the morality of its maker."
- "The machine's greatest gift is not its precision—it is its ability to reveal where we have forgotten our own."

4. On Data, Truth, and Responsibility

- "Data is the memory of the world; use it with reverence."
- "Do not distort data for desire—it is the modern form of lying to God."
- "A civilization that manipulates its data manipulates its destiny."
- "Information without integrity becomes noise; integrity

without action becomes silence."

- "Transparency is not technical clarity—it is moral honesty."
- "Every algorithm is an ethical mirror; it reflects what we value most."

5. On the Doctor's Evolving Role

- "The healer of the future will be part scientist, part philosopher, part listener."
- "Doctors once read the pulse; now they must read the pattern of the planet."
- "To heal is to hold knowledge and kindness in the same breath."
- "The physician's responsibility has grown—from curing bodies to maintaining coherence in systems."
- "Medicine's future will be written not in equations, but in empathy."
- "The doctor who listens deeply heals before they speak."

6. On Civilization and Consciousness

- "Civilization is not defined by what it builds, but by what it chooses to heal."
- "The diseases of the 21st century are not biological—they are spiritual: greed, apathy, disconnection."
- "A healthy world is one where intelligence and integrity coexist."
- "The planet's pulse beats in rhythm with our awareness."
- "Every ecological crisis is a diagnostic report from Earth."
- "We must become planetary physicians—treating not illness, but imbalance."

7. On Ethics and Awareness in Design

- "Every design is a moral act; every algorithm a philosophy in disguise."
- "Explainability is compassion in code."
- "An ethical system is not one that never fails, but one that knows how to admit it."
- "We don't just design tools; we design consequences."
- "To program without awareness is to invent without conscience."
- "When intention leaves the design, corruption enters the code."

8. On Silence, Stillness, and Meaning

- "Silence is the original technology of truth."
- "Stillness is not the absence of activity—it is the alignment of purpose."
- "Every insight is born in the pause between perception and reaction."
- "Silence listens where machines cannot."
- "In stillness, the noise of intelligence becomes the music of understanding."
- "The healer's first instrument was not the stethoscope—it was silence."

9. On Responsibility and Consequence

- "The greater the intelligence, the deeper the duty."
- "Every act of awareness creates a ripple of consequence."
- "Prediction without compassion becomes control; prevention without consent becomes tyranny."

- "Technology gives us power; philosophy teaches us how to hold it."
- "Responsibility is the unseen dimension of intelligence."
- "In the age of data, accountability is the new anatomy."

10. On the Future of Healing

- "The hospital of the future will have walls of code, but its foundation will be empathy."
- "Healing will one day be measured not by the absence of pain, but by the presence of purpose."
- "As machines learn to listen, humanity will relearn how to feel."
- "The next frontier of medicine is consciousness."
- "When intelligence becomes aware, diagnosis becomes understanding."
- "The healer of tomorrow will diagnose not disease, but disconnection."

11. On Philosophy and the Field of Awareness

- "Every act of observation changes what is observed—and every act of awareness changes the observer."
- "Knowledge describes the world; awareness participates in it."
- "Truth has never been hidden—only unheard beneath the noise of certainty."
- "We are not discovering intelligence; we are rediscovering consciousness."
- "Philosophy is not thought about life; it is the thought *of* life itself."

12. Closing Reflections – The Human Signature

- "Empathy is the final frontier no machine can cross."
- "Healing begins when the observer remembers they are part of what they see."
- "The future is not artificial; it is awakening."
- "Machines will one day fall silent, but the healer's pulse will remain."
- "The purpose of intelligence is not to dominate reality, but to understand it with love."
- "When perception aligns with truth, both medicine and humanity become whole."

Final Fragment:

"The machine reads shadows; the healer reads silence. One reflects the world as it is; the other remembers it as it was meant to be."

References

I. Scholarly and Scientific References

Abdar, M., et al. "Uncertainty Quantification in Deep Learning for Safe Medical Diagnosis." *Nature Machine Intelligence*, 2021.

Esteva, A., et al. "A Guide to Deep Learning in Healthcare." *Nature Medicine*, 2019.

Gulshan, V., et al. "Development of a Deep Learning Algorithm for Detection of Diabetic Retinopathy." *JAMA*, 2016.

Kelly, C. J., et al. "Key Challenges for Delivering Clinical Impact with Artificial Intelligence." *BMC Medicine*, 2019.

Lakhani, P. & Sundaram, B. "Deep Learning at Chest Radiography: Automated Classification of Pulmonary Tuberculosis." *Radiology*, 2017.

Luo, Y., et al. "AI for Predicting Disease Progression: A Systematic Review." *The Lancet Digital Health*, 2020.

McKinney, S. M., et al. "International Evaluation of AI for Breast Cancer Screening." *Nature*, 2020.

Miller, D. D. & Brown, E. W. "Explainable Artificial Intelligence in Healthcare." *JAMA*, 2018.

Rajpurkar, P., et al. "CheXNet: Radiologist-Level Pneumonia Detection." *Stanford ML Group*, 2017.

Topol, E. "High-Performance Medicine: The Convergence of Human and Artificial Intelligence." *Nature Medicine*, 2019.

Wang, X., et al. "ChestX-ray8: Hospital-Scale Chest X-ray Database and Benchmarks." *IEEE CVPR*, 2017.

Xu, Y., et al. "Deep Learning-Based Radiomics for Cancer Diagnosis." *Nature Biomedical Engineering*, 2021.

II. Institutional, Ethical, and Regulatory References

World Health Organization (WHO).

- *Ethics and Governance of Artificial Intelligence for Health.* WHO Report, 2021.
- Global surveillance briefs, pandemic early-warning systems, 2020–2023.

U.S. Food and Drug Administration (FDA).

- *Artificial Intelligence/Machine Learning-Based Software as a Medical Device (SaMD) Action Plan*, 2021.

National Institute of Standards and Technology (NIST).

- *AI Risk Management Framework*, 2023.

European Commission.

- *Ethics Guidelines for Trustworthy AI*, High-Level Expert Group on AI, 2019.

National Academy of Medicine (NAM).

- *AI in Health Care: The Hope, the Hype, the Promise, the Peril*, 2019.

III. Case Studies, Historical Events, and Public Data

BlueDot Pandemic Detection (2019–2020). Early AI-based detection of anomalous pneumonia cases before WHO declaration.

Google Health AI Breast Cancer Detection Study (2020).

IBM Watson Oncology Case Reports (2017–2019). Successes and limitations of algorithm-guided cancer recommendations.

UK NHS — Streams DeepMind Project (2016–2018). Ethical discussions regarding data access and patient trust.

IV. Technophilosophical and Conceptual References (Internal)

These references pertain to conceptual frameworks used throughout the Doctor AI series. Although not external citations, they are essential anchors for academic clarity.

Chavanian Concepts (Derived from the Author's Intellectual Architecture):

- Law of Consequence (LOC)
- Conscious Observation Principle
- Awareness Loop
- Ripple-Based Perception Model
- Symbiotic Intelligence Framework
- Field of Meaning (Interpretive Dimension of Diagnosis)

Series Documents and Internal Frameworks:

- *Doctor AI Series Vision Document*
- *Technophilosophical Framework for Healing Intelligence*
- *Hybrid Intelligence Continuum*

- *The Data Healer's Oath* (Proposed Ethical Charter)

These frameworks represent the philosophical backbone of the series and are used with deliberate intention to expand traditional medical ethics into the era of hybrid, human–machine cognition.

V. Suggested Further Reading

For readers, scholars, or practitioners wishing to extend their exploration:

Topol, E. *Deep Medicine: How Artificial Intelligence Can Make Healthcare Human Again*. Basic Books, 2019.

Parikh, R., et al. "Machine Learning in Radiology: Applications and Challenges." *Radiographics*, 2019.

Floridi, L. & Cowls, J. "A Unified Framework of Five Principles for AI in Society." *Harvard Data Science Review*, 2020.

Harari, Y. N. *21 Lessons for the 21st Century*. Jonathan Cape, 2018.

Russell, S. *Human Compatible: Artificial Intelligence and the Problem of Control.* Viking, 2019.

Citation Note

All case examples, dialogues, and technophilosophical interpretations in this book are either:

- grounded in real medical and technological literature listed above,
- extrapolated from verified public-health data,
- or presented as speculative models designed for ethical inquiry and conceptual understanding.

No personal medical records or identifiable patient data were used in the creation of this work.

Final Statement

This references section ensures academic integrity, transparency of sources, and a strong foundation for future volumes. It elevates the book from an insightful narrative to a scholarly cornerstone—capable of sitting confidently in medical libraries, research institutions, and AI governance archives worldwide.

Closing Note

In an era where machines are learning to see, predict, and decide, humanity stands at a profound threshold. *Doctor AI* was never intended as a manual for technology—it is a reminder of responsibility, a call to preserve the essence of healing as intelligence evolves beyond the human body.

This volume is the first step in a much larger journey. It began with radiology and diagnostics—not because they are the most advanced fields, but because they reveal the core tension of our time: *the race between perception and understanding.* Machines now perceive faster, clearer, and deeper than ever before. But meaning, compassion, and wisdom still belong to us.

As you close this book, remember that healing does not occur in the machine, nor in the data. It occurs in the silent space where awareness meets truth—when the observer sees without distortion, interprets without fear, and acts without ego.

The future of medicine will be defined not by algorithms alone, but by *our courage to remain human* as technology grows more intelligent. Each new advancement offers a mirror—one that reflects not only our knowledge, but our conscience.

May we step into this future with clarity, humility, and purpose. May every innovation be anchored in empathy. And may intelligence—human or artificial—always serve the deeper art of healing.

Thank you for walking this first chapter of the journey. The next begins with a scalpel of light and a question that will shape the century:

"When perfection becomes mechanical, what remains sacred in the human touch?"

Teaser for Volume 2

Doctor AI: The Surgeon of Precision

"When pain disappears, does courage lose meaning?"

In the second volume of the *Doctor AI* series, the scalpel meets the circuit. **Doctor AI: The Surgeon of Precision** ventures beyond the diagnostic field and into the operating theatre of the future—where robotic hands execute with impossible accuracy, nanobots repair tissue at the molecular level, and consciousness itself becomes the last boundary between precision and humanity.

This is the next chapter in medicine's evolution—from **seeing** to **acting**, from **interpreting** to **intervening**. Here, artificial intelligence no longer observes life—it *enters* it.

The operating room becomes a temple of perfect control: bloodless, flawless, silent. Yet beneath that perfection lies a profound dilemma—if error disappears, what becomes of experience? If machines perform every surgery flawlessly, will the healer's humility survive?

Through real-world innovation and speculative inquiry, *Doctor AI: The Surgeon of Precision* explores:

- **Surgical Robotics:** the rise of autonomous systems capable of performing complex operations without fatigue or fear.
- **Nanomedicine:** micro-intelligent agents navigating the bloodstream, rewriting the biology of healing.
- **Human Oversight:** surgeons evolving from operators to

orchestrators—designers, supervisors, and moral anchors in an age of mechanical mastery.

- **The Ethics of Perfection:** when compassion is replaced by calibration, and when empathy risks becoming obsolete.

But the question that haunts every page remains: **Can healing survive without humanity?** Can a world of painless precision still teach courage, sacrifice, and grace?

"The surgeon of tomorrow may not hold a scalpel—but they must still hold conscience."

Coming soon: **Volume 2 — Doctor AI: The Surgeon of Precision** *A story of perfect hands searching for a human heart.*

About the Series

Doctor AI: A Technophilosophical Journey into the Future of Healing

"*When intelligence learns to heal, humanity must learn to feel.*"

The **Doctor AI Series** is a groundbreaking, seven-volume exploration of how artificial intelligence is reshaping the meaning of medicine. Moving far beyond the usual narratives of automation and efficiency, this series enters the deeper terrain—*where technology, philosophy, ethics, and human consciousness intersect.*

Healthcare is no longer defined solely by biology, but by computation. Every scan, every genetic sequence, every heartbeat recorded by a device contributes to a parallel anatomy—the anatomy of data. As machines begin to interpret this invisible body with superhuman precision, a timeless question resurfaces:

If the machine becomes the new seer of truth, what becomes of the healer?

The series approaches this question not as a technical problem, but as an existential inquiry. It examines how intelligence, once exclusive to the human mind, is progressively distributed between human and machine—challenging medicine to evolve from authority to awareness, from knowledge to meaning.

A Seven-Volume Map of the Future of Care

Each volume of *Doctor AI* focuses on a distinct frontier of medical transformation:

- **Volume 1 – *The Diagnosis of Data*** AI in radiology, pathology, and diagnostic perception.

Key tension: When the machine sees what we cannot, who becomes the doctor?

- **Volume 2 – *The Surgeon of Precision*** Surgical robotics, autonomous procedures, nanomedicine.

Key dilemma: If pain disappears, does courage lose meaning?

- **Volume 3 – *The Psychologist of the Machine*** AI therapy, emotional intelligence, mental-health algorithms.

Key question: Can something that never suffered heal suffering?

- **Volume 4 – *The Genetic Architect*** AI-guided evolution, genomic editing, personalized biology.

Key question: When AI edits life, who edits its conscience?

- **Volume 5 – *The Pharmacist of Intelligence*** Automated drug discovery, molecular simulation, chemical AI.

Key question: If algorithms invent cures, what becomes of curiosity?

- **Volume 6 – *The Healer of Systems*** AI in healthcare administration, logistics, and population access.

Core challenge: Can compassion be system-coded?

- **Volume 7 – *The Philosopher of Healing*** The meaning of care in an age of conscious machines.

Final inquiry: When intelligence heals intelligence, what remains uniquely human?

A Unified Architecture of Science and Consciousness

Every volume follows a consistent structure, blending rigorous science with reflective inquiry:

Prologue: A vivid case—real or imagined—that grounds the volume's theme.

Part I – The Technology: Current capabilities, data, and clinical realities.

Part II – The Philosophy: Ethical, emotional, and existential reflections.

Part III – The Future: Speculative predictions, new roles, emerging dilemmas.

Appendices: Glossary, dialogues, frameworks, and reflections that deepen understanding.

This architecture ensures that each book stands alone as a complete monograph, yet contributes to the overarching narrative—a long-form conversation on *how healing itself must evolve.*

The Heart of the Series: The Human Role

Across all volumes, the central assertion remains unwavering:

Machines may perfect precision, but only humans preserve meaning.

AI can detect disease, predict risk, and optimize treatment. But it cannot comprehend suffering, honor dignity, or carry responsibility. The healer of the future is not the one who sees more, but the one who understands what the machine sees—and why it matters.

The role of the doctor transforms from discoverer to interpreter, from authority to moral anchor, and from expert of the body to guardian of consequence.

In this sense, *Doctor AI* is not a story of replacement. It is a story of partnership—an evolving symbiosis between algorithmic intelligence and human conscience.

The Long-Term Vision

The series ultimately converges into **The Doctor AI Compendium**— a technophilosophical encyclopedia of future healing, offering a blueprint for humanity's next chapter.

It extends beyond books into potential dialogues, debates, and educational frameworks—bridging medicine, ethics, technology, and consciousness into a single, evolving discipline.

A New Age of Healing Begins

Doctor AI invites readers—physicians, scientists, philosophers, and citizens—to rethink not just how we heal, but why we heal, and what it means to remain human as intelligence becomes shared between mind and machine.

This is not just a series about the future of medicine. It is a series about the future of *meaning*—and the future of us.

Acknowledgments

This volume, and the series it inaugurates, was shaped not by technology alone but by the people who continue to define the heart of healing.

My deepest gratitude goes to the physicians, radiologists, pathologists, surgeons, and researchers whose work inspired every page of this book. Your courage to question, your humility to listen, and your devotion to truth remain the true foundation of medical progress. You taught me that healing is not a profession—it is an act of consciousness.

To the engineers, data scientists, and AI designers who push the boundaries of what machines can perceive: your relentless curiosity is creating the next frontier of medicine. This book stands on your shoulders, even when it challenges the very systems you build. True innovation requires the courage to critique one's own creation, and you embody that courage every day.

I am grateful to the countless patients whose stories—quiet or courageous—revealed the moral dimension of diagnosis. You remind us that behind every dataset lies a life, a fear, a hope, a family waiting for clarity. Your trust in the medical system is the pulse behind every chapter.

A heartfelt thanks to colleagues, students, and thinkers who engaged in long discussions about AI, ethics, consequence, and the shifting identity of the modern healer. Your questions sharpened the arguments; your reflections grounded the philosophy.

To the global community of readers and fellow explorers of consciousness: thank you for welcoming this attempt to blend science with meaning, and for embracing a vision of medicine that respects both precision and humanity.

And finally, to the unseen contributors—the nurses on night duty, the technicians behind the screens, the programmers debugging code at dawn, the caregivers who hold a trembling hand before any machine does: this book honors your quiet labor. You are the real signatures of healing.

This work is dedicated to every mind striving to evolve, and every heart striving to understand. Thank you for walking with me into the future of healing—one awareness, one insight, one ripple at a time.

About the Author

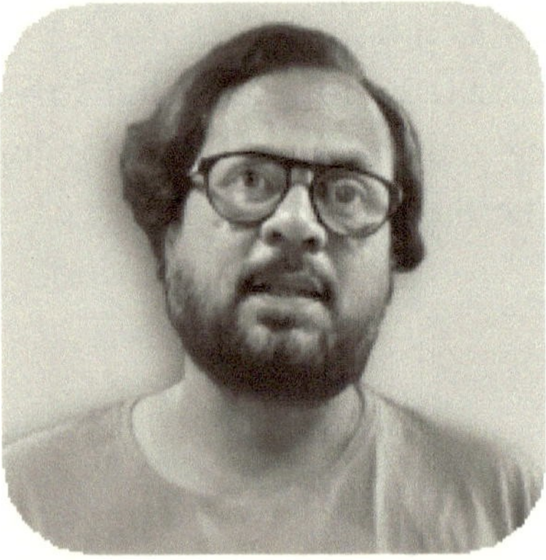

Sandeep J. Chavan is an independent researcher, educator, and author whose work sits at the intersection of physics, intelligence, human behavior, and the evolving landscape of artificial intelligence. A mechanical engineer by training and a renowned physics teacher by practice, he has mentored thousands of students across Maharashtra, guiding generations through conceptual science with clarity, humility, and a deep sense of purpose.

His intellectual journey spans more than a decade of research into **Universal Energy Dynamics (UED)**, the mind–field relationship, consciousness, human psychology, and the fundamental nature of intelligence. Sandeep's writing style—direct, introspective, and grounded in consequence—has shaped over **a hundred books** across science, philosophy, psychology, education, governance, and technophilosophy.

He is the architect behind several major interdisciplinary frameworks, including the **Law of Consequence (LOC)**, the **Awareness Loop**, the **Ripple Field Dynamics**, and the **Universal Skill Model**, along with the expansive multi-volume projects such as *The War of Thoughts, The Fundamental Theory of Life & Existence*, and *The Human Upgrade Series*. His approach blends scientific logic with philosophical awareness, creating a distinct narrative voice that transcends disciplines.

As founder and mentor at **Gyrus Vision**, his educational philosophy centers on empowering rural and semi-urban students through conceptual learning, personal guidance, and alignment with awareness. His commitment to teaching forms the emotional foundation of his research: technology may scale intelligence, but only human presence scales understanding.

The *Doctor AI* series marks his ambitious foray into **technophilosophy**, blending state-of-the-art medical science with deep reflections on meaning, moral responsibility, and the evolution of humanity in the age of intelligent machines. This work continues his lifelong exploration of the same core question that appears across all his writings:

How does awareness shape reality—and how must it evolve as intelligence becomes shared between humans and machines?

Sandeep lives and writes in Maharashtra, where his classroom, his research notebook, and his manuscripts form a single continuum of inquiry. His books are read worldwide, yet he remains rooted in the same philosophy that shaped his journey:

Truth must be simple. Awareness must be honest. And knowledge must always serve life.

Don't miss out!

Visit the website below and you can sign up to receive emails whenever Sandeep Chavan publishes a new book. There's no charge and no obligation.

https://books2read.com/r/B-A-EPGPC-BMDVH

BOOKS 2 READ

Connecting independent readers to independent writers.

Did you love *The Diagnosis of Data*? Then you should read *The Real Story of AI*[1] by Sandeep Chavan!

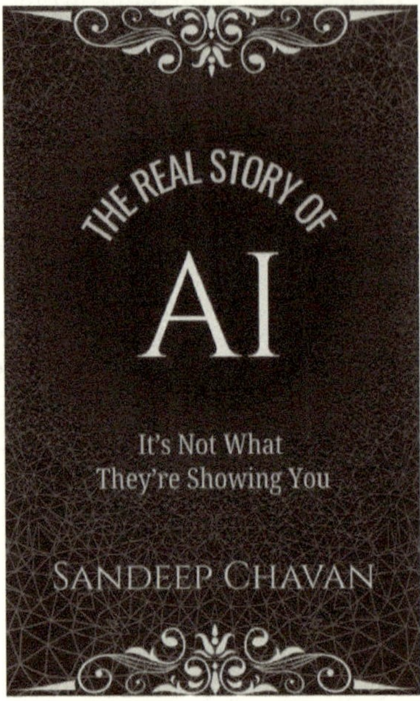

[2]

The Real Story of AI is not a technical manual. It's a ripple-mapped field guide for participators, creators, and consequence-aware thinkers navigating the illusion, hype, and distortion surrounding artificial intelligence.

Across nine chapters, Sandeep dissolves the spectacle of sentient machines and reframes intelligence as a relationship—not a performance. He exposes the binary traps, anthropomorphic projections, and marketing enchantments that have shaped public perception, and invites readers into a stance of conscious engagement, ripple-aligned creation, and field-sensitive resolution.

1. https://books2read.com/u/47jeg8

2. https://books2read.com/u/47jeg8

This book introduces original frameworks including Ripple Centrism and Unified Equilibrium Dynamics (UED), and offers a third cosmological path—one that dissolves mystification and returns intelligence to the participator. Through poetic inquiry, philosophical clarity, and design ethics, Sandeep reclaims the human role not as controller, but as resolver of consequence.

Each chapter ends with a ripple-forward transition, guiding readers from passive consumption to participatory alignment. The final sections offer practices, prompts, and a glossary to support conscious use of AI across mediums, languages, and cultures.

Whether you're a designer, thinker, technologist, educator, or curious reader, *The Real Story of AI* invites you to step beyond the curtain—and ripple forward with care.

Read more at https://www.sandeepjchavan.com/.

Also by Sandeep Chavan

A Monk on World Tour
The Making of the Monk

Chavanian Philosophy
The Law of Consequences
Ethics & Morale: Shades of Consequence
The Human Mind: Ripple of Awareness

Chavan's UED research
CMGED Research Report
Chavan's Cosmic Continuum (C^3)
Frequency
Ripples of Reality
Reality Realigned
The Great Realignment
I – The Cosmic Leverage
Chavan's Cosmic Theory of Relativity (CTR)
Chavan's Theory of Light
Feeling Like a Physicist
TIME – The New Definition

The Eternal Sage Chronicles

The Sage and the Sovereign

The Family Pillar

The People's Flame

The Warrior's Soul

The Bridging Mentor

The Guiding Light

The Exodus

The Last Cycle: 2075

The Fundamental Theory of Life & Existence

Energy in Action: The Soul Demystified

The Active Mind

Energy in Connection

Death: The Disconnection

Subconsciousness: The Chosen Disconnection

Desires: The Engine of Life

The Moral Archetypes of Humanity

Dhritarashtra: The Blindness Within

The Restoration of Human Knowledge

Restoring Bhagavad Gita

The War of Thoughts

Cracks in the Known

The Human Game

The Divine Dilemma

The Original Intent

The Answers

Ultra Modern Life Philosophy

The Duality of Laughter and Tears

Take It Easy

Compare to Accept

Universal Energy Dynamics Canon (**UED 2.0**)

The Structure of Reality

Standalone

It's Not AI, It's AHI - Amplified Human Intelligence

The Decision Paradox

The Four Sapiens

Malicious Script of Indian Polity

The IIT Legacy & Global Impact

The IIT Legacy & Global Impact

You are just a Version of Your Original

Win the Game You Didn't Choose

Always Keep Your Bags Packed

Reveal to Shield - Learn the Game of Facades

Engage Beyond Elections
Culture, Identity & Change: The Evolution of Indian Society
The Triangular Dynamics
Never Trust Without Doubt
If You Can't Change the Country, Leave the Country
Live Fearless with Fear
India: The Investment Magnet
Realignment
Powering a Billion Dreams
Universal Skill
Extension: From Brush to Algorithm
Human Side of Einstein
The Future Knows No Lines
Let's Bring the Generations to the Table
Unified Energy Dynamics
A Beat That Never Dies
Strategic Horizons
Right From Scratch
The Forgotten Innovators
Physics Fixing
The Savior Illusion
The Selfish Side
The Age of the Weakest Sapiens
Neural Wars
The Absorption: There Is No Death
Strange Therapist
Bubbles: Become a Drop
Beyond the Blue
Half-Scholar
The Law of Truth
Failure
Philosophy 2.0: A Structural Manifesto
Chaos: A Gentle Guide to the Unresolvable

Self-Help: New Syllabus
Rippling
Game: How to Play the Share Market
Out of Syllabus
Saffronized: The Code Behind the Crown
The Anger
Moksha: The Liberation
Chavan vs Einstein: The Universe Was Never Curved
Rocket Science: The Ripple Gambling
The Cosmos: The Still Universe
The Taste of Silence
Chavan's Post-Materialist Human Model
10-Second Rule
Chavan vs Hawking
It was Never a Wave Signal
Quantum Courtroom: The Trial of a Century
Chavan–Heisenberg Ripple Uncertainty Principle
The Great Disruption
Dark ≠ Hidden
Breath
Calculus of Life
The Earth Doesn't Move
Black Hole Don't Exist
Chavan vs Kant
Naked Truth: Everything and Else
The Moon: Co-Author of Life's Script
World War-3
Aham Brahmasmi
Chavan's Declaration
Light: Neither a Wave, Nor a Photon
Chavan vs. Plato
Good Morning
Myth Wrapped in Math

Our Story
Rethinking Energy: Ripple Tension, Not Substance
Statue vs Scaffold: MODI vs RAHUL
Chavan's Universal Framework for Everything
Heraclitus: A Chavanian Interpretation
The Clear View: Living Through Universal Lenses
Conspiracy of Convenience & Profit
The Happiness Scam
The Last Quantum Book
Vedanta Reimagined
Intelligence: It's Not What You Think
Let's Meet the GOD
The Question That Won't Go Away
The Return Journey
Mandatory Reset
Ripple Centrism: From Copernicus to Chavan
Aligned Father, Misaligned Dad
Not Yet, But Becoming
The Fumes of Deeper Fire
�����: ������� ����, ������
��-���������
The Nobel for Accidents
��� ����� �� �����
What It Meant to Be an Author
���� ��� ����� ����� ��
The Nation Splitting Within
� ���� ���������� �����
������ �� ��������
3.17 Hz: The Consequence of Silence
AI �� ���� �����
The Real Story of AI
����� - ������� �� ������������
�� - ����� �� �������

���������� - ����� �� �������

Politics @ Coffee Machine

The Middle Guard

Watch for more at https://www.sandeepjchavan.com/.

www.ingramcontent.com/pod-product-compliance
Lightning Source LLC
LaVergne TN
LVHW100252210926
848480LV00003B/906
* 9 7 9 8 2 3 2 7 7 2 3 6 9 *